LIVING TO BE

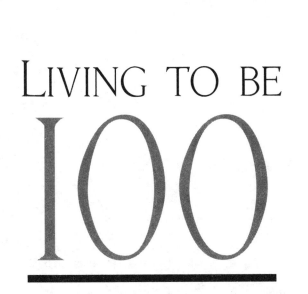

100

16 Common Lifestyle Characteristics of the Oldest and Healthiest People in the World

BY MICHAEL E. HOWARD, PH.D

BIOMED GENERAL • CONCORD, CA • ©2012

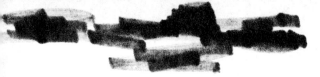

LIVING TO BE 100

ISBN 978-1-893549-18-0

Biomed General
P.O. Box 5727
Concord, CA 94524-0727
USA

925.288.3500 *main*
925.680.1201 *fax*
info@biocorp.com

Author
Michael Howard, Ph.D.

Editors
Richard Colman, Ph.D.
Mary O'Brien, M.D.

Cover Art and Layout
Nancy Loquellano

This book is not designed to substitute for professional medical advice. Always consult a medical professional before making major changes in eating habits or taking supplements.

To obtain more information about Biomed General's products and services, please contact us at the above address.

ABOUT BIOMED GENERAL

Biomed General is an organization that provides health care professionals with the latest scientific and clinical information. Biomed's live seminars and home-study courses are designed to help health professionals provide better care for their patients. Biomed General operates nationwide in the United States as well as internationally.

Biomed General
P.O. Box 5727
Concord, CA 94524-0727
USA
925.288.3500 *main*
925.680.1201 *fax*
info@biocorp.com

About the Author

DR. MICHAEL HOWARD is a board-certified clinical neuropsychologist and health psychologist who is an internationally-recognized authority on brain-behavior relationships, traumatic brain injury, dementia, stroke, psychiatric disorders, aging, forensic neuropsychology, and rehabilitation.

During his 30-year career, Dr. Howard has been on the faculty of three medical schools, headed three neuropsychology departments, and directed treatment programs for individuals with brain injury, dementia, addiction, chronic pain, psychiatric disorders, and other disabilities. He currently lectures throughout the United States and abroad on these topics and on his current areas of research, which include life expectancy and successful aging, disease prevention, physical and mental fitness, and stress management.

Dr. Howard currently resides in Texas and is a consultant lecturer, author, and researcher for the *Academy of Biotechnology, Institute for Natural Resources,* and *Biomed General Corporation.*

TABLE OF CONTENTS

> *Centenarians are the navigators who have successfully completed a long, perilous voyage. Somehow, this one relatively small group of people has nimbly negotiated the maze of maladies, mishaps, and military conflicts that commonly lead to death. Not only do they escape death, but by and large they escape ill health for most of their lives. And, as we have found, their experience has much to tell us about how to live, too.*
>
> —THOMAS PERLS, MD, MPH, ET AL.
> *Living to 100: Lessons in Living to Your Maximum Potential at Any Age*

> *The calculus of aging offers us two options: we can live a shorter life with more years of disability, or we can live the longest possible life with the fewest bad years. As my centenarian friends showed me, the choice is largely up to us.*
>
> —DAN BUETTNER
> *The Blue Zones: Lessons for Living Longer From the People Who've Lived the Longest*

Most of us want to live as long as we can—to be 100 years old and beyond. The older we get, the more important this seems to be. We also want to keep functioning well when we reach old age. In other words, we want to live long but not get old! Well, believe it or not, that can happen, and it's happening more often than ever before. There are now a large number of people in the world more than 100 years old, and many of them are functioning remarkably well mentally, physically, and emotionally. How do they do it? Is it inherited? Is it luck? No, as you will find out by taking this course, it is mostly our lifestyle choices—not just our genes—that determine how long and how well we live. Want to know what these oldest old people have done to allow them to live so long and so well? Want to know if you can do this, too? Want to make it to be 100 years old and still have a vital and healthy life? This course explores these questions and some of the possible answers.

People who live to be 100 years old and older are called *centenarians.* Having a lot of them around is a pretty new thing. No one knows how many people made it to 100 years of age prior to the beginning of recorded history (about 5,000 years ago), but the numbers were probably extremely small. Centenarians are still somewhat of a rarity even today, but the percentage of the population who make it to 100 years old has dramatically increased in the past 200 years (Vaupel and Jeune, 1995; Wilmoth, 1995).

Research in the area of human longevity has increased steadily in recent years, and empirical information about the select group of centenarians and supercentenarians (those living to be 110 years and older) is growing rapidly. This research has found that both genes and lifestyle factors play a role in extreme longevity. However, as will be seen, lifestyle characteristics appear to be the most important predictors of a long and healthy life. By studying centenarians in many areas of the world, we now have some

There are now a large number of people in the world more than 100 years old, and many of them are functioning remarkably well mentally, physically, and emotionally.

valuable insights into how someone can construct a lifestyle of positive health practices that will significantly increase the chances of joining this select group of "oldest old" (Vaupel et al, 1998; Vaupel and Jeune, 1995; Lehr, 1991; Poon et al, 1997; Perls, 2004; Perls et al, 1999; Wilmoth, 1995).

Do we really want to increase our life spans if we are doomed to eventually be frail and demented for many years? What most of us want is a long and *healthy* life. Many people, even some researchers, believe that most of the oldest old are decrepit and disabled and have miserable lives. The field of geriatrics, unfortunately, seems to focus on what's wrong with old people and how bad aging is. Reading some of the geriatrics literature can lead to the idea that the final years of life are awful, dominated by illness, disability, and physical frailty. Is this the way it really happens? It is true that one-third of Americans die before age 65 years? Only half of us will make it to 78 years, and many who live this long have disabling chronic diseases. So, is disabling illness the fate of centenarians? Get ready for a very pleasant surprise.

The two dozen or so ongoing studies of centenarians around the world paint a very different picture of the oldest old. These people not only live a long, long time but also seem to avoid, endure, or delay the age-related disabling illnesses that affect most of us. In fact, a large percentage of centenarians are amazingly mentally,

Lifestyle characteristics appear to be the most important predictors of a long and healthy life.

emotionally, and physically intact. Studies show that about two-thirds of people who are 100 years old and older will delay, if not completely escape, the common age-related diseases. A smaller proportion will survive for many years to centenarian status even after developing these age-related diseases (Evert et al, 2003). These longest-living people in the world are teaching us that growing older does not necessarily mean growing sicker.

About a third of the oldest old live independently, and another

> **These people not only live a long, long time but also seem to avoid, endure, or delay the age-related disabling illnesses that affect most of us.**

20 percent or so seem to have the capacity to do so even if they are in assisted living settings. That means one-half of centenarians have the mental and physical capacity to live independently. In fact, studies such as the New England Centenarian Study have found that many 100-year-olds are markedly healthier than the average 70- to 80-year-old. The Georgia Centenarian Study reported that more than 60 percent of its participants claimed that their health had *improved*

in the previous five years since their 90s. Instead of finding out what's wrong with the oldest old, centenarian studies have, amazingly, found out what's *right* about them!

Centenarians are a group of people who seem to possess genetic, environmental, and lifestyle attributes—plus maybe some luck—that allow them to live to very old age by either surviving, delaying, or avoiding the common age-related diseases and disabilities that shorten most lives. The attributes that most strongly predict who will live to be 100 years of age are becoming clear through research, and are outlined in this course. These predictors appear to be mostly lifestyle factors. Can you plan and live a lifestyle that will increase your odds of reaching centenarian status and still be healthy, vigorous, and happy? The answer is *yes*, it appears you can.

What does it take to live a long and healthy life? How much does diet, exercise, and lifestyle matter? What is the quality of life among the oldest old? Answers can be found by looking at the two dozen centenarian studies being conducted around the world.

An analysis of these studies shows that there are about 16 physiological and lifestyle markers that characterize people who become centenarians. Constructing a lifestyle incorporating these 16 characteristics can increase your odds of becoming a healthy and happy 100-year-old. You will see that these are simple things that all of us can do. Describing the 16 steps to become a centenarian is the focus of this course. Before we get there, however, some background information on life expectancy and life spans may help put all this in perspective.

Centenarians are a group of people who seem to possess genetic, environmental, and lifestyle attributes—plus maybe some luck—that allow them to live to very old age by either surviving, delaying, or avoiding the common age-related diseases and disabilities that shorten most lives.

❀ ❀ ❀ ❀ ❀

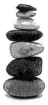

A Short History of Life Expectancy: From the Stone Age to the Information Age

Life expectancy is lengthening, driven by new knowledge and prevention in heart disease, cancer, and other diseases, as well as improvements in public hygiene, standards of living, nutrition, and other factors of modern life.

—THOMAS PERLS, MD, MPH, ET AL.
Living to 100: Lessons in Living to Your Maximum Potential at Any Age

Life expectancy is the number of years that a person can expect to live. This number has increased dramatically in developed countries of the world in the last 200 years or so. In the Neolithic Stone Age, just 13,000 years ago, the average life expectancy was about 25 to 30 years. Infant mortality, early childhood injuries and disease, and childbirth trauma in women resulted in early deaths for many people. Physical trauma and bacterial and viral illnesses claimed many lives. However, although starvation was a significant threat to survival for early hunter-gatherers, the average human in the Stone Age was rather well-nourished, and neither malnutrition nor starvation was a common condition or cause of death. Nevertheless, at that time in human history, only a very few individuals lived into their 80s or 90s. During the Stone Age, it is estimated that only one in 10 people ever made it to 60 years of age, so getting to 100 was extremely rare, if it happened at all.

How about those stories of ancient people living several hundred years or so? Are they accurate? Yes and no. There are well-known Biblical accounts of a number of ancient individuals who were reported to have lived for an extraordinarily long time. Methuselah, for example, the Hebrew patriarch and grandfather of Noah, lived 969 years according to the Book of Genesis (5:27). He reportedly died in the year of the Great Flood. How could it be that someone could live 969 years when life expectancies were so short? Probably because a common method of calculating age at that time was the lunar numeric system. Age was often measured in those ancient times by monthly lunar cycles, not the solar cycles that later became the basis for the Julian calendar. By this method, 969 lunar cycles would make

Methuselah 78 years old when he died. In those times, that was a very, very old age indeed.

From the Agricultural Revolution about 12,000 years ago until the year 1600 AD, the average European life expectancy hovered between 20 and 24 years. This is shown clearly by European skeletal remains of people from early Mediterranean agricultural societies through the Egyptians, Classical Greeks, Romans, and Dark Ages (Wilmoth, 1995; Vaupel & Jeune, 1995). While some areas of the world may have had longer or shorter average life expectancies, the overwhelming evidence from worldwide studies of human remains over the last 10,000 years shows that the average life expectancy for most people until very recently was less than 25 years. This life expectancy was shorter than the 25 to 30 years found in Stone Age remains. Why? There are a number of reasons. Malnutrition was certainly a major cause of disease and death as agricultural diets became very limited to fatty meats, grains, and dairy products. Micronutrient variety declined tremendously when agricultural peoples no longer consumed the wide variety of fruits, roots, vegetables, and nuts that hunter-gatherers did. Agricultural people didn't get the variety of vitamins, minerals, and other key micronutrients that their Stone Age predecessors did. Because of this, diseases of micronutrient deficiencies such as scurvy and beri-beri appeared. Living close to animals and to each other resulted in escalating rates of communicable infectious diseases between animals and humans such as tuberculosis. Epidemics of communicable diseases, which never existed in the scattered hunter-gatherer populations, became a major threat to life as people lived close together in one place.

> **Until about 400 years ago, it was rare that anyone could live to 100 years of age.**

For most of recorded history, beginning about 5,000 years ago, until about 400 years ago, the average human did not live very long. One reason is that the death curve in European and early American agricultural societies was a "skewed left" type of pattern, where there were very high death rates in early childhood. As in hunter-gatherers, infant mortality and early childhood diseases and trauma remained major threats to survival in early agricultural societies, skewing the average life expectancy downward.

Getting to five years of age was a struggle, with some studies suggesting that only one in four Stone Age children lived to their fifth birthday. If, however, a child did make it to five years of age, many lived past the age of 25 years. Ancient historical accounts of famous people show that a number of them prior to the year 1600 may have made it into their 70s. However, examination of remains suggest that the common citizen probably had a much shorter life expectancy than the more well-to-do—pulling the average way down. In any case, until about 400 years ago, it was rare that anyone could live to 100 years of age because of the multiple threats to life that existed during the last 10,000 years agricultural societies have existed.

In the last 400 years—and the last 200 years in particular—things have changed. In most of the developed countries of the world, human longevity has dramatically increased. In the year 1800 in the United States, when John Adams was turning over the presidency to the third president, Thomas Jefferson, life expectancy was about 37 years. This would be about 10 years longer than most Romans lived. But, by the year 1900, the average American life expectancy had jumped to 47.3 years—a remarkable 10-year jump in just a century.

Even more astonishing, American life expectancy is now about 78 years—nearly doubling in the past 100 years. This dramatic leap in life expectancy in such a short time is unprecedented in human history. Why has this happened? The answer appears to be nature, not nurture. Our genetic code has not changed much at all. Instead, rapid environmental and lifestyle changes in developed countries, especially during the last 100 years, have been the main cause of much longer human life spans.

> **Rapid environmental and lifestyle changes in developed countries, especially during the last 100 years, have been the main cause of much longer human life spans.**

The numbers of Americans in older age groups are markedly higher than they were just 100 years ago. The 85-years-old-and-older group is now the fastest-growing segment of the American population (Hetzel and Smith, 2001). The pattern of the U.S. population has markedly changed from being "bottom-heavy," with the majority of people under

20 years of age, to where all age groups from zero to 80+ years old are roughly the same size (Perls et al, 1999). By the year 2020, it is estimated that one of six Americans will be over the age of 65 years—the same number that will be under the age of 20 years. This "graying of America" and the corresponding leap in numbers of centenarians is having—and will have—an enormous impact on our culture.

> **Three *"ations"* have played a big part in the large 20th and 21st century increases in life expectancy: *medication, vaccination,* and *sanitation.***

What environmental conditions have recently changed to explain increased longevity? For one thing, it appears that changes in the three *"ations"* have played a big part in the large 20th and 21st century increases in life expectancy: *medication, vaccination,* and *sanitation.* Just 100 years ago, infectious diseases like pneumonia, tuberculosis, and enteritis/diarrhea/dysentery were the three leading causes of death in the U.S. With the widespread development and use of antibiotics in the 1900s, bacterial illnesses that led to short life expectancies have largely been controlled and even eradicated in developed countries. Bacterial diseases have now been replaced by chronic disorders of old age as the main causes of death. The leading causes of death in the U.S. are now heart disease, cancer, stroke, chronic obstructive pulmonary disease, and diabetes. These are all chronic diseases with advancing age being a significant risk factor. Advances in treatments for these chronic diseases in the last 50 years or so have helped increase both average life expectancies and the numbers of centenarians. Most centenarians still die from heart disease, but they would have died much sooner had it

> **Bacterial diseases have now been replaced by chronic disorders of old age as the main causes of death.**

not been for medications that control cholesterol levels and blood pressure. Recent health-enhancing changes in clean drinking water, food purity, and prevention of maternal and childhood deaths have also played a big role in increasing longevity in industrialized countries such as the United States.

NATIONAL DIFFERENCES IN LIFE EXPECTANCY: THE "LONGEVITY GAP"

Do Americans live the longest? No. In fact, we are 48th on the list of the world's countries in longevity. Countries like Okinawa, Singapore, Hong Kong, Japan, and Switzerland are way ahead of us, all living an average of 83 years and longer. Where you live and the lifestyle you choose, as well as genetics, have the greatest effects on life expectancy. For example, there are about 225 sovereign countries and protectorates in the world. Among them, the people of Okinawa have the longest average life expectancy of about 84 years. Many of the countries who have the longest life expectancies are in the Pacific Rim and around the Mediterranean Sea. On the other hand, the inhabitants of many countries have much shorter life spans. The so-called *longevity gap* between the life expectancies of the longest-lived people in some countries and the shortest-lived people in other countries is huge—50 years! If you are born in sub-Saharan countries like Botswana and

> It is *where* you are born and *how* you live your life that makes the greatest impact on how long and how well you will live.

Lesotho, the average individual only makes it to 35 years of age. This fact alone should dispel the belief that most of successful aging is genetic. We all belong to the species *homo sapiens*, with similar genetic influences on life expectancy. It is *where* you are born and *how* you live your life that makes the greatest impact on how long and how well you will live. As might be expected, the countries with the longest average life expectancies tend to have the highest percentage of centenarians, while the countries with the lowest life expectancies have the fewest centenarians.

How Many Centenarians Are There?

As life expectancies have increased around most of the world in recent years, the number of centenarians has skyrocketed. The proliferation of centenarians is a very new development in human history. In Ancient Egypt, 5,000 years ago, probably less than one in a million made it to 100 years of age. Some longevity experts have said that the incidence of centenarians before 1900 may have been as small as one per century. Other researchers think that, in many small countries such as Denmark, there may have been no centenarians at all before the 1800s. Compared to a yearly one percent growth in the general population in industrialized countries, the centenarian group is increasing by eight percent per year. In the year 1900, only one in 100,000 Americans was a centenarian. Today, 100 years later, they are 10 times as common—one in every 8,000 to 10,000.

In particular, the past several decades have seen a huge jump in the numbers of centenarians in the world (Terry et al, 2008). In 1953, there were fewer than 200 centenarians reported living in France, but there are 3,000 reported today. In industrialized nations across the world, one in 10,000 people now reach 100 years of age, and this incidence may double in just a few years (Perls, 2006). Out of six billion people in the world, there are now about 300,000 or so centenarians. The highest percentage appears to be in Okinawa, a group of 44 inhabited islands that stretch 800 miles between Japan's main islands and Taiwan and a prefecture of Japan, whose inhabitants also have the longest life expectancy.

The Okinawan Centenarian Study has studied the group of oldest old in this country for the last 30 years. Since there has been a national birth and death registration system for the last century in Okinawa, it is known that there are currently about 700 centenarians out of a population of 1.3 million—about 54 per 100,000. This may be the highest percentage of centenarians in a national population in the world, and is about five times the number found in most industrial countries.

Countries vary a great deal in their number of centenarians, which is usually related to the average life expectancy of the country or region. Documented centenarians in countries with low overall life expectancies, such as some in sub-Saharan Africa, are very rare.

In the U.S., there are now more than 70,000 centenarians, and the numbers are increasing rapidly each year.

In the U.S., there are now more than 70,000 centenarians, and the numbers are increasing rapidly each year. The exact number is difficult to determine with certainty because there was no national birth registration system in the U.S. until 1940. The number of centenarians varies by state in the U.S., with the largest percentage of centenarians being in South Dakota, followed by Iowa. By 2050, there may be more than 800,000 Americans over 100 years of age.

Having such large numbers of people becoming centenarians is unprecedented in human history and is largely a result of 20th century changes in health practices.

How Long Can We Live?

There is an limit to how long a human being can live. Each year someone lives over the age of 100, the chance they will make it to their next birthday drops dramatically. Getting from age 100 to age 110 years—a *supercentenarian*—is difficult. Among the 300,000 centenarians around the globe, the Gerontology Research Group and the Supercentenarian Research Foundation have documented only 86 supercentenarians in the entire world—78 women and eight men. Making it to 120 years of age borders on the near impossible, and may be the outside limit of our species' current maximum life span. At the present time, there are no known individuals in the world who are older than 120 years of age. Has anyone ever made it to 120 years of age? The answer is yes, but it's a very small club with only one known member.

❀ ❀ ❀ ❀ ❀

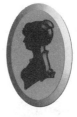

2

**Who Has Lived the Longest?
A Good Bet: It Was a Woman**

The longest human lifespan where birth and death could be formally documented by birth and death certificates was that of a woman. She was a Frenchwoman named Mme. Jeanne Louise Calment, who died in France in 1997 having lived 122 years and 164 days (Allard, Lebre and Robine, 1994). She was born on February 21, 1875 and died on August 4, 1997. To help get your head around how long this interesting woman lived, she was born when Ulysses S. Grant was President of the United States and she died when Bill Clinton was President. She was born in Arles, France and lived there for all of her life.

Mme. Calment became well-known in France at age 115 when it was discovered that she was the last living person to have met the Impressionist painter Vincent Van Gogh. He had visited her father's fabric store to buy some canvas when she was 13 years old.

(She described him as crass, dirty, badly dressed, and thoroughly unpleasant.) Mme. Calment's family members also lived to advanced ages: her brother lived to the age of 97 years, her father to 93 years, and her mother to 86 years. She outlived both her daughter and grandson. Marrying a wealthy store owner at age 21 years, she never had to work, but led a very active lifestyle, pursuing hobbies like tennis, cycling, swimming, roller skating, piano, and opera. She took up fencing at age 85 years, and reportedly rode her bicycle regularly until age 100 years.

Jeanne Calment was an exception to individuals who have some of the usual lifestyle characteristics that predict who will reach centenarian status. For example, she smoked until age 117 years and consumed two glasses of wine per day for most of her life. When asked for the secret to living to such an old age, Mme. Calment ascribed it, on one occasion or another, to garlic, vegetables, red port wine, cigarettes, avoiding brawls, two pounds of chocolate per week, and olive oil, which she liberally poured on all her food and rubbed into her skin. She had a marvelous sense of humor and was famous for her frequent one-liners.

Mme. Calment lived on her own until shortly after her 110th birthday, when it was decided she should move to a nursing home. She remained in good shape and was able to walk until she fractured her femur and required surgery due to a fall at age 114 years 11 months.

The next longest-lived person whose birth and death can be documented was a woman who was 119 years old when she died. Many women have been documented as living 115 years or longer. The oldest living man whose life span can be documented in recent history was either 112 or 115 years old when he died—there is some dispute here. It would appear, when it comes to numbers, that women win the longevity race.

❀ ❀ ❀ ❀ ❀

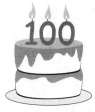

Yes. Around the world, women centenarians outnumber men about nine to one. In most American studies, approximately 85 percent of women and 15 percent of men make it to 100 years of age, a ratio of about six to one. Only about one male in 20,000 reaches the age of 100 years in the U.S. compared to six women.

In all developed countries and in most developing ones, women have a longer life expectancy than men. Currently, most studies find that the average American woman will live to about 81 years of age and the average man to about 75 years old. That's about a six-year life expectancy difference. However, when men and women live to older ages, the gap narrows. On average, American women over the age of 65 years will outlive their male counterparts by only three years or so, and the gap is narrowing. The sex ratio in the

65 years old and older category increased from 67 men per 100 women in 1990 to 70 men per 100 women in the year 2000. The older one gets, the closer the average life expectancies between the sexes becomes. Of those Americans who make it to 75 years of age, the average woman only outlives the average man by two years. However, centenarians are a big exception to this closer life expectancy. Worldwide, women are nine times more likely to make it to 100 years of age than men. Despite some exceptions (for example, male centenarians outnumber women on the Mediterranean island of Sardinia), the percentage of women who make it to 100 years old in most areas of the world is markedly higher than that of men.

Why do women live longer than men? Why do women centenarians in most countries typically outnumber the guys nine to one? The effects of estrogen, menstruation-related toxic elimination, the extra x chromosome, less job stress, better disease survival, and higher levels of social behavior and social support have all been thought

Around the world, women centenarians outnumber men about nine to one.

to play a role. Evidence also suggests that part of the advantage women have in reaching 100 years old may be longevity-enabling genes that maximize the length of time during which women can bear children (Perls and Fretts, 2001; Perls et al, 1999). Clearly, this trait would be beneficial since having children later in life would require more longevity to raise them. Interestingly, the New England Centenarian Study found that women who have a child in their 20s and another in their 40s were much more likely to make it to 100 years old than a woman who had two children in her 20s.

When it comes to the number of centenarians in nearly all areas of the world, women have a big advantage over men. When quality of life is taken into account, however, there is a reversal of fortune. In an interesting contrast, men centenarians are actually healthier than women, are less frail; have better mental abilities; are less likely to develop dementia, such as Alzheimer's disease, at the highest age levels, and more likely to live independently (Ozaki et al, 2006; Perls, et al, 1993, 1999; Terry et al, 2008). It appears that women have better functioning than men in younger old age but men, although fewer in number, have better functioning than women in extreme old age. This may be because men must be in excellent health and/or functionally independent to achieve such extreme old age (Perls et al, 1999). Women, on the other hand, may be better at being physically and socially able to live with chronic and often disabling health conditions and age-related diseases at the oldest ages. The New England Centenarian Study found that about two thirds of male centenarians are non-disabled and can do their activities of daily living independently, while only about 40 percent of female centenarians can (Terry et al, 2008). The Georgia and Japanese Centenarian studies also found more men than women are capable of living independently (Ozaki, 2006).

❀ ❀ ❀ ❀ ❀

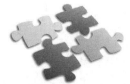

4

Becoming A Centenarian:
Stone Age Genes vs. Industrial Age World

It was during the Old Stone Age, which began some three
million years ago, that our body chemistry nearly reached its
current stage of development...the way our bodies function
is virtually unchanged from those who lived hundreds of
thousands of years ago but our lifestyle is vastly different.
Since the Agricultural Revolution began about 12,000 years
ago, the discordance between our genetic blueprint and our
lifestyle has accelerated. The result is a biological disaster...
Life was short for those who lived during the Stone Age because
of diseases that modern medicine, with a strong assist from
modern plumbing, has almost totally eliminated. However,
their nutritional health was excellent. The health challenges
that we encounter now are almost entirely of our own doing.

—PHILIP J. GOSCIENSKI, M.D.
Health Secrets of the Stone Age: What We Can Learn from Deep
in Prehistory to Become Leaner; Livelier; and Longer-Lived

Human bodies and brains today do not significantly
differ genetically from humans who lived in the
Stone Age as nomadic hunter-gatherers at the end of
the Neolithic period 13,000 years ago. Put a suit on a
guy from the Stone Age and a dress on a Stone Age
woman, and they'd look just like us. We are the same
as they were—but the environment that we live in is

not the same. Therein lies the problem. Our world has changed dramatically in the last few hundred years, but our genes have not. Our human genetic code is designed to protect us from threats to the survival of our species that existed 13,000 years ago—threats that no longer exist for most of us in modern America, such as starvation, dying of thirst, and animal predators. Our genetic code has not had time to adapt to the drastic cultural and environmental changes of the modern world. Now, the major threats to health and life in America are largely due to a mismatch between our Stone Age genes and the lifestyle of the Technological and Information Age we live in. Genes that saved our lives and our species in the Stone Age have become major threats to our lives now. As will be seen, the trick to surviving to a very old age involves creating a lifestyle that resembles that of our Stone Age ancestors, while taking advantage of the health benefits from modern

> **Our world has changed dramatically in the last few hundred years, but our genes have not.**

medicine, dentistry, and sanitation that protect us from potentially fatal diseases.

FROM STARVATION TO OVEREATING

Our bodies are genetically designed to protect us from the Stone Age threat of starvation. The main daily activity of the Stone Age person was finding food. There was no agriculture or food storage. During the Stone Age, the nomadic hunting and gathering lifestyle did not always result in food being found. It was feast or famine. Therefore, our bodies are designed to go three or four weeks without food. Our fat cells, called *adipocytes*, are marvelously genetically engineered to store triglycerides as energy so this could be utilized when we went days without eating. We are also designed to feel pleasure in the brain when our stomachs are full of food, called *satiation*. Those who ate the most when food was found stored the most fat and were protected against starvation. In addition, our brains experience pleasure when three senses of taste are stimulated: sweet, fat, and salt. These tastes were rare in the Stone Age environment, but two of them, sweet and fat, are responsive to food very high in needed calories, and the other, salt, helped us store water and maintain critical metabolic balances. These genetic pathways helped our species survive 13,000 years ago.

The Stone Age diet varied day-by-day and was different in different regions of the world. Mostly, we ate fruits, vegetables, roots, tubers, and nuts, with occasional lean meats, fowl, and fish. With the dawn of the Agricultural Revolution about 12,000 years ago, our diets markedly changed. We began to consume larger amounts of grains, dairy products, and fatty red meats. In agricultural cultures, food became relatively plentiful, and some cultures actually had an overabundance of food. Unfortunately, our bodies have no genetic protection against today's abundance of food and the pattern of overeating seen in industrialized nations. We eat to satiation again and again on a diet full of high-calorie processed foods that are stuffed with addictive sweet, fat, and salty tastes that stimulate excessive consumption. We have no effective genes that protect against an abundance of food—especially lots of the kinds of foods we aren't designed to eat. The same genetic pathways that prevented us from starving in the Stone Age now cause obesity, diabetes, and cardiovascular disease, three of the greatest threats to our lives. As will be seen, two of the 16 steps to get to 100 years old involve playing to our Stone Age genes by eating fewer calories and maintaining low blood sugar.

From Activity to Inactivity

Our bodies are genetically designed to be active and undergo daily physical exercise. Our Stone Age genes are designed for a body that walked six to 22 miles per day in search of food, water, shelter, and social contacts. Even our ancestors who became farmers after the Agricultural Revolution were very physically active. However, with the advent of the Industrial Revolution in the mid-1800s and the Technology and Information Age in the late 1900s, the human labor-saving devices we have invented and mass-produced have caused human activity levels to drop precipitously. Today, only about one in five Americans exercises regularly. Lack of exercise is a major contributor to the leading causes of death in the U.S. The lack of energy expenditure in the form of exercise coupled with a high-calorie diet is the main reason two thirds of Americans are either overweight or obese. Lack of exercise may be the one single greatest cause of shortened life expectancies in the U.S., because inactivity is such a powerful risk factor for obesity, diabetes, cardiovascular disease, and even Alzheimer's disease. As might be expected, getting regular exercise—like our Stone Age genes are programmed for—is one of the 16 steps to get to 100 years old.

From Acute Stress to Chronic Stress

Our brains are still designed to go into stress mode every once in a while when confronted by a threat such as a predator or starvation. We are genetically designed to mount a "flight-or-fight" *acute* stress response to seeing a saber-tooth tiger looking for his lunch. Unfortunately, our brains and bodies were never constructed to cope with the *chronic daily stress* in our current world from a raging boss, financial problems, rush-hour traffic, or looking at the mess in your teenager's bedroom (Sapolsky, 1998). We can deal effectively with occasional acute stress, but we do not have genetic pathways to cope with chronic stress.

Chronic stress leads to disabling mental and physical illnesses that shorten life expectancy. Continued bombardment of the brain by stress leads to significant emotional problems such as anxiety disorders, anger, insomnia, and depression. These disabling disorders are also powerful risk factors for developing hypertension, heart disease, stroke, diabetes, and Alzheimer's disease. It's easy to see why reducing stress and achieving a calming serenity are two of the 16 steps to become a centenarian.

FROM DEHYDRATION TO HYPERTENSION

In the Stone Age, one of the great threats to humans was dehydration and dying of thirst. When engaged in strenuous activity, we can go only about three to four days without water. Our bodies are genetically constructed to utilize sodium and hormones to hold on to water in our bodies. Now, with high levels of sodium consumption and plentiful water, this is a genetic recipe for hypertension—one of the greatest threats to health and life. Cardiovascular disease—heart disease and stroke—is the biggest killer of American men and women, and hypertension is one of the biggest risk factors for cardiovascular disease. It is no surprise, then, that one of the 16 steps to get to 100 years old is to eat a mostly vegetarian diet, such as the Mediterranean diet, which happens to be low in sodium.

From Clotting Wounds to Cardiovascular Disease

In the Stone Age, we moved about a great deal in a world full of threats to body integrity. Cuts, lacerations, and bites were common in hunter-gatherer cultures, and are even to this day. Those of us who had excellent blood clotting with high levels of clotting factors like fibrinogen and thromboxane were able to clot blood in wounds, prevent infections, and avoid bleeding to death. Effective blood clotting helped us survive in the world of 13,000 years ago. However, in our current industrialized world, the single event that will kill the greatest number of Americans is a clot that forms in one of the coronary arteries or cerebral arteries, i.e., a heart attack or stroke. This is a very new phenomenon. Just 100 years ago in the U.S., cardiovascular disease was not a common cause of death. Now, it's our biggest health threat. In 2009, heart disease and stroke killed as many Americans as the next five leading causes of death put together. The blood clotting genes that used to save our lives are now killing us because of our dramatically changed environment and lifestyle. It's no surprise that reducing the risk of cardiovascular disease by lowering blood pressure and blood cholesterol are another two of the 16 steps to becoming a centenarian.

To Become an American Centenarian: Avoid Cardiovascular Disease and Cancer

Centenarian studies show that making it to 100 years of age usually means having a generally healthy lifestyle and avoiding, delaying, or surviving the modern causes of death that shorten life. The main causes of death for human beings have changed greatly over the past few centuries and even the past few decades. Infectious diseases were the primary reason for short life expectancies. From the time of Julius Caesar, about 2,000 years ago, until the early 1900s, infections

> **Making it to 100 years of age usually means having a generally healthy lifestyle and avoiding, delaying, or surviving the modern causes of death that shorten life.**

from bacteria and viruses were the major killers. For example, eight of the 10 leading causes of death in the United States in 1860, about the time the Civil War started, were infectious diseases: tuberculosis, diarrhea, cholera, pneumonia, diphtheria, dysentery, scarlet fever, and nephritis.

More Americans died in the Civil War than in any other war we have ever been in. What do you think the leading cause of death was for soldiers of both the North and South in that hailstorm of rifle bullets and artillery shells? Dysentery.

In 1900, when the average life expectancy in the U.S. was 47.3 years, pneumonia and tuberculosis were still the leading causes of death, and about 90 percent of the population died from infections. All that has changed since the Scottish scientist Alexander Fleming discovered penicillin in 1928 and modern medicine began to control infectious diseases with antibiotics. Now, only three to four percent of people in the developed world die from bacterial infections, one of the main reasons we have longer life expectancies.

So, what are the biggest threats to our lives in modern America? The leading causes of death in the U.S. have changed a lot in the last century. The Centers for Disease Control and Prevention (CDC) found that the 10 leading causes of death in 2003 (the last data compiled) were as noted in the table above (CDC National Vital Statistics Reports, No. 13, April 19, 2006).

Reducing the risks for the top 10 causes of death is the key to a long and healthy life.

The causes listed in *Table 1* are responsible for 1,913,000 people dying each year in the United States—80 percent of all deaths. There are about 100,000 diseases listed in the *International Classification of Diseases-10*, but there is very little for most of us to worry about from the bottom 99,990 of them. Reducing the risks for the top 10 causes of death is the key to a long and healthy life. In fact, reducing the risks for the top three, heart disease, stroke, and cancer, is by far the most important since they account for nearly 60 percent of all deaths in the U.S.

Table 1. *Leading Causes of Death in 2003*

Rank	Cause	Percentage %
1	Heart disease	28
2	Cancer	23
3	Stroke	6
4	Chronic obstructive pulmonary disease (COPD)	5
5	Accidents	4
6	Diabetes	3
7	Influenza and pneumonia	3
8	Alzheimer's disease	3
9	Kidney disease	2
10	Septicemia	1

What are the controllable risk factors for the 10 most deadly diseases? Not surprisingly, they are high cholesterol, high blood sugar, high blood pressure, poor diet, tobacco use, lack of regular exercise, being overweight or obese, chronic stress, depression, and drinking too much alcohol. It is also no surprise that the opposites of all seven of these factors are included among the 16 common lifestyle characteristics of centenarians. Avoiding the risk factors for the 10 leading causes of death is key to having a very long and healthy life.

Table 2. *Hierarchy of Mortality in Men and Women, 2003*

Men	Women
1. Heart disease	1. Heart disease
2. Cancers	2. Cancers
3. Stroke	3. Stroke
4. Accidents	4. COPD/emphysema
5. COPD/emphysema	5. Diabetes mellitus
6. Diabetes mellitus	6. Influenza & pneumonia
7. Influenza & pneumonia	7. Alzheimer's disease
8. Suicide	8. Accidents
9. Kidney diseases	9. Kidney diseases
10. Liver disease & cirrhosis	10. Septicemia

There are some gender differences in the top 10 causes of death in the U.S. As shown in *Table 2*, men and women have a somewhat different hierarchy of mortality (National Vital Statistics Report, 2003, Vol. 50, Tables 1 and 2).

There are gender differences both within and between these causes of death. For example, Alzheimer's disease is a greater risk for women, and dying from accidents is a much bigger problem for men. More men die of tobacco-related cancers than women because they smoke more, but women are catching up as their smoking rates have risen in recent years. More women die from chronic obstructive pulmonary disease (COPD), which is also usually smoking-related.

> **For both men and women, the single biggest obstacle to making it to 100 years old is cardiovascular disease.**

Heart disease and stroke are numbers one and three causes of death for both men and women. Although men are more likely to have a heart attack or stroke, women are more likely to die of these diseases. For both men and women, the single biggest obstacle to making it to 100 years old is cardiovascular disease. Heart disease and stroke kill about as many Americans as the next five leading causes of death combined. As noted by the cardiologist Scott Grundy (quoting Sir William Osler), "You are as old as your arteries." (Grundy, 1999). If your arteries are stiff and clogged with cholesterol, you are not likely to live a long time.

It is important to understand that avoiding cardiovascular disease involves mostly lifestyle choices, *not* genetics. The INTERHEART study of

29,000 people in 52 countries found that lifestyle risk factors predicted

Avoiding cardiovascular disease involves mostly lifestyle choices, *not* genetics.

90 to 94 percent of all heart disease, the leading cause of death for Americans (Salim et al, 2004). Genetics accounted for less than 10 percent of the risk.

Cancer is the second leading cause of death in the U.S., and it is also a largely preventable disease. Researchers from the Harvard School of Public Health found that at least 65 to 80 percent of cancers could be prevented by implementing some fairly simple healthy lifestyle choices. Nearly 95 percent of diabetes is type 2 diabetes, largely caused by lifestyle factors such as obesity, high-fat and high-calorie diets, and lack of exercise. Designing a lifestyle that lowers the risk for heart disease, stroke, cancer, and diabetes is a major key to long and healthy life. These lifestyle factors are included in the 16 steps to increasing the chance of living to 100 years and beyond.

❀ ❀ ❀ ❀ ❀

5   A Long Life Span or a Long Health Span: Which Do You Want?

> *"When old age descends upon you,*
> *slowness of movement appears;*
> *The eyes become dim; the ears hard of hearing;*
> *Muscles become weak, every movement is difficult;*
> *And the spirit is forgetful*
> *and cannot even remember yesterday."*
>
> —Ptahhotep

Does getting old sound like fun? The above description was written by Ptahhotep, a physician and advisor to the Pharoah Izezi of Egypt 4,600 years ago. He was describing himself. Back then, the average Egyptian lived about 25 years or so. Ptahhotep, however, wrote that just before he died, when he was older than 100 years. Although from his description, old Ptahhotep seems to be falling apart, a very high percentage of centenarians are actually healthy, happy, physically intact, and mentally sharp for nearly all their lives. Ptahhotep himself had evidently stayed remarkably cognitively and physically intact until just a brief period before he died. In other words, he had a long "health span."

When asked, most people will say that they want a long *life span*, but that may not be what most of us really want. Since most Americans will have some years of disability at the end of their lives when they consider their quality of life to be poor, what we really want is probably a long *health span*. This is the length of time from birth until we become disabled. Studies show that many centenarians have remarkably long health spans with vigorous functioning over nearly all their lives—staying relatively healthy until becoming significantly sick or disabled only a short time before their deaths (Perls et al, 1999). This is especially true for the subgroup of centenarians who are still living independently at age 100 years (Ozaki et al, 2006; Poon 1992).

When it comes to centenarians, older does not necessarily mean sicker. There is a common myth that all of the very old are doddering and dependent. However, studies have found that about 25 to 30 percent of centenarians still live independently, are cognitively intact, and generally vibrant and full of life at age 100 years (Perls, 2004; Poon et al, 1992). Even more of the centenarians—around 72 percent of the males and 34 percent of the females—score in the independent living range on tests of activities of daily

Many centenarians have remarkably long health spans with vigorous functioning over nearly all their lives.

living, such as the Barthel Index, even though some of them may live in retirement or assisted-living centers. Remarkably, some studies have found more than 40 percent of *supercentenarians* (110 years old or older) to be independent or require minimal assistance in their activities of daily living (Schoenhofen et al, 2006). So, fully one-half of centenarians are still cognitively and physically healthy enough to be able to live independently—pretty amazing. Of course, that still leaves about 50 percent who have some form of dementia (maybe 25 percent with significant dementia), and about 60 to 70 percent with at least some level of disability, some of whom some are completely dependent (Hagberg et al, 2001; Samuelsson et al, 1997). However, even those who developed significant dementia by 100 years of age had delayed the onset of any significant mental impairment until at least an average age of 92 years—well beyond the average life expectancy of most Americans (Perls, 2004). Even centenarians with demonstrated neuropathological markers of Alzheimer's disease often do not show significant mental deficits in the form of dementia—suggesting the existence of a "cognitive reserve" in these oldest old that protects their brains (Perls, 2004).

Individuals who have reached 100 years of age seem to have avoided or resisted the effects of the common age-related diseases that occur in people between their 50s and 90s. According to New England Centenarian Study findings, centenarians have managed to either survive (called "survivors"), delay ("delayers"), or escape ("escapers") the common causes of death that kill people at older ages (Evert et al, 2003).

Some—"survivors"—develop heart disease or other chronic diseases before the age of 80 years, but survive them without having significant levels of disability (loss of functioning) until just before death.

This is called *compression of disability*. This may be the key prerequisite for most people making it to 100 years of age (Terry et al, 2008). Nearly one-third of centenarians live with diagnosed age-related diseases or morbidities for 15 or more years. Studies of Danish centenarians found that 72 percent of them had some level of cardiovascular disease, 60 percent had urinary incontinence, 54 percent had osteoarthritis, and 51 percent had dementia. And yet, these "survivors" were still alive and functioning at 100 years of age. In the New England Centenarian Study, about 24 percent of male centenarians and 43 percent of females were survivors of 10 major age-related diseases. So, the oldest females are twice as likely to be survivors of age-related illnesses as the oldest males.

"Delayers" have typically lived relatively healthy lives without serious disorders of cognitive, emotional, and physical functioning until very late in life. Studies show that about 95 percent of American centenarians are functionally independent at age 92 years, with low rates of mental illness and depression (Perls et al, 1999; Perls, 2006). They usually stay healthy throughout their lives before becoming seriously sick or disabled for a short period just before dying. This is called *compression of morbidity*, with morbidity being age-related diseases. In 424 centenarians aged 97 to 119 years in the New England Centenarian Study, about 44 percent of male centenarians and 42 percent of females were delayers (Evert et al, 2003).

"Escapers" seem to completely avoid the typical diseases of aging (Bernstein et al, 2004). These individuals, in remarkable physical and cognitive shape at 100 years of age, comprise about 23 percent of males and 15 percent of female centenarians. Thus, nearly two-thirds of centenarians have either delayed or escaped significant age-related morbidities. For some reason, although females are much more likely to be centenarians, males over 100 years of age are much more likely to be escapers of any disabling disease of aging and have better cognition and physical functioning than their female counterparts (Terry et al, 2008).

❀ ❀ ❀ ❀ ❀

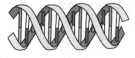

It is well known that people who live long and stay well often have relatives who had long and healthy lives. Making it to 100 years of age does run in families; becoming a centenarian is much more likely if your parents did. Even if they didn't make it to 100 years old, they were more likely to have shortened life spans due to smoking and not receiving optimal medical care and vaccinations. So, they might have had the genes to have longer life spans and been successful, if they had practiced healthier habits and had more access to medications.

Studies of children of centenarians show a tremendous benefit from genetic longevity, especially in a lower risk for cardiovascular disease—the main killer of Americans (Terry et al, 2004). As noted by Dr. Dellara Terry, the Director of the Genetics of Longevity Study

People who live long and stay well often have relatives who had long and healthy lives.

at Boston University Medical Center, "Children of persons who have reached 100 years of age are less likely to have cardiovascular and other chronic diseases." Compared to matched control subjects at age 72 years, offspring of American centenarians had 78 percent lower risk of heart attack, 83 percent lower risk of stroke, and 86 percent lower risk of developing diabetes mellitus—three of the five leading causes of death for Americans (Adams et al, 2008). Overall, these offspring of centenarians were 81 percent less likely to die by age 72 years than control subjects of the same age.

Having a sibling who makes it to 100 years old is also a great genetic advantage for longer life. Siblings of Okinawan centenarians were found to live an average of 11.8 years longer than matched controls (Willcox BJ et al, 2005; 2006). Studies show that 100-year-olds are four times as likely to have a sibling who lived past age 90 years than the average American. Compared to siblings of non-centenarians, male siblings of centenarians were at least 17 times as likely to reach 100 years old themselves, and female siblings were at least eight times as likely to do so (Perls et al, 2002). Perls and colleagues have recently identified over 100 genes that appear to increase the chance of having very long and healthy lives.

However, this may not all be due to genes. Traits that run in families are not all genetic. Families often share the same activity levels, eating habits, and other environmental and lifestyle factors that can influence health and longevity. Other familial biological factors can also affect aging. For example, female children of younger mothers are more likely to make it to 100 years old than those born to older mothers. On the other hand, women who have children in middle age are about four times more likely to become centenarians than those who have children in their 20s (Perls, Alpert & Fretts, 1997). Birth order may also be important. Studies have shown that first-born children, especially women, may be more likely to reach 100 years old than later-born siblings.

So, how much of human longevity is due to genes? Studies of the genetic effect on human life span have not been able to estimate a number or percentage regarding the power of genes to push us to age 100 years. However, many studies have found that genetic determinants are a powerful force in predicting who does and does not reach old age (Perls et al, 1999). The effects of genes on aging may be even greater in those who live to the extremes of old age. Unfortunately, there is not much we can do at this time about the genetic factors that affect successful aging. You'll either inherit good aging genes or you won't. It's a roll of the DNA dice.

It is not known exactly which or how many genes are involved in helping us reach the oldest ages. It appears that there are a number of genes that may be involved in either extending life or slowing the aging process in both humans and animals, and researchers have identified a few of these. For example, the manipulation *(genetic engineering)* of the SIRT gene, has lengthened the lives of fruit flies and mice by as much as 35 to 50 percent. In humans, an area on chromosome four, as well as genes that regulate the synthesis of proteins and control cholesterol, may affect longevity. Variation in the gene FOXO3A has a positive effect on life expectancy in humans and has been found much more often in people living to age 100 years. A study by Takata and colleagues in a 1987 *Lancet* article found Okinawan centenarians to have genetic polymorphisms in the HLA (human leukocyte antigen) that appeared to give them a lower risk for life-shortening inflammatory and autoimmune diseases. Also, centenarians appear to have very low levels of a particular gene, Apolipoprotein E e4, which is known to be a genetic risk for Alzheimer's disease and a shorter life expectancy. The e2 variant of this gene is associated with lower levels of serum cholesterol, and apolipoprotein B and was found more frequently than the e4 variant in studies of Japanese, French, and Finnish centenarians (Hirose et al, 1997). Even the telomeres, the ends of the chromosomes that shorten with each cell division and promote cellular apoptosis or suicide, appear to be longer in centenarians and indicate a genetically-induced slower aging of body cells (Terry et al, 2008). So, many genes and gene mutations are known to be associated with very long life spans.

Being lucky enough to have avoided life-shortening genetic diseases such as Huntington's disease certainly helps in making it to 100 years of age. Genes also play a role in many other fatal diseases like cardiovascular disease, cancer, and diabetes. Thomas Perls, MD, MPH, who heads the New England Centenarian Study, says that if you've managed to side-step genes for fatal diseases, "there's nothing stopping you from living independently well into your 90s."

However, genes aren't all that matters in successful aging by a long shot. Heart disease is the single biggest obstacle to making it to 100 years old, and the INTERHEART study found that that lifestyle factors, not genetics, predicted 90 to 94 percent of all heart disease. A landmark 1981 study concluded that diet plays a significant role in most cancers, including as much as 90 percent of the risk for stomach and colon cancer. Tobacco smoking accounts for more than 90 percent of lung cancers and strongly contributes to heart disease and stroke.

The large increases in the numbers of centenarians argue against genetics being the largest factor in having a long life. In Okinawa, for example, there were only 32 documented centenarians in 1976, but in 2006 there were 560. Such a recent increase far exceeds the overall population growth and is not due to genetic changes in a 30-year period of time. Environmental and lifestyle changes must be involved in some way. It's not just in Okinawa. Environmental and lifestyle changes appear to have dramatically impacted recent increases in longevity and numbers of centenarians in many parts of the world.

Many people believe that factors such as socioeconomic status, access to health care, and whether or not someone has health insurance are the largest factors involved in life expectancy. Actually, these and things like how much money is spent on health care do not play a major role. As C.J. Murray and colleagues (Murray, Kulkami, & Ezzati, 2005) found, when determining why Americans have long lives, factors like exercise, smoking, drinking alcohol, blood pressure, blood sugar, and blood cholesterol are far more important in determining how long the average American lives than whether someone has health insurance or access to health care. Prevention of disease seems to be more important than treatment of disease in determining who gets to 100 years old (Danaei et al, 2009; Danaei et al, 2010). As found in studies of independently-living centenarians such as the Japanese Centenarian Study, good health practices and lifestyle choices throughout life play the most important role in having a long life with (1) preserved cognitive abilities, (2) good psychosocial status, and (3) the ability to do activities of daily living (Ozaki et al, 2006).

> **Certain environmental and lifestyle conditions can interact with good aging genes to profoundly affect the chance to reach 100 years of age.**

Dr. Thomas Perls believes that we are genetically capable of living to at least 85 years of age, but that the lifestyle choices can alter this number drastically in either direction. Certain environmental and lifestyle conditions can interact with good aging genes to profoundly affect the chance to reach 100 years of age. What are these environmental and lifestyle factors?

If you have followed what has been said so far, you can already see several commonalities among the various centenarian groups around the world.

❁ ❁ ❁ ❁ ❁

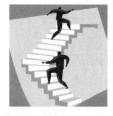

 7

The 16 Steps to Make it to 100 Years of Age

Average life expectancy should be 85, and it would be 85, if more people would take disease prevention seriously at a time when it is still possible to make an impact, and maintain good health habits for a lifetime. Unfortunately, the vast majority of baby boomers do a terrible job of preparing for old age. High-fat diets, smoking, excessive drinking, and lack of exercise not only reduce people's chances of achieving older age, they markedly increase the likelihood of a longer period of poor health in a shorter life. Yet many of us probably have the genes to get to old age and perhaps extreme old age. We just have to learn how to use them.

—Thomas Perls, MD, MPH, et al.
Living to 100: Lessons in Living to Your Maximum Potential at Any Age

If you live the average American lifestyle, you may never reach your potential maximum lifespan. You might even fall short by as much as a decade. But what if you could follow a simple program that could help you feel younger, lose weight, maximize your mental sharpness, and keep your body working as long as possible?.... While these practices are only associated with longevity and don't necessarily increase it, by adopting them, you'll be adopting healthy habits that should stack the deck in your favor.

—Dan Buettner
The Blue Zones: Lessons for Living Longer From the People Who've Lived the Longest

How do centenarians avoid life-ending diseases for so long? What characteristics do they share that seem to make them resistant to disease? What methods can be utilized to extend life and reach 100 years of age? These questions have intrigued us throughout history, and many methods to extend life have been practiced through the ages—with varying results. About 2,000 years ago in India, for example, people ate gold dust to extend life. At about the same time, the Chinese believed that eating a powder made from gold, sulphur, jade, mercury, and lead would lead to a long life (one wonders how many of these folks made it past 50 years eating that stuff!). King David of Israel had an even more interesting take on extending life: he believed that you would live long if you prayed and inhaled the breath of young girls (which was a common belief in those ancient times). Even as recently as the late 1800s, a prominent European physician injected himself with a mixture of dog and guinea pig testicles to prolong life. Needless to say, there is little evidence that any of these rather diverse practices to extend life ever worked.

Other ancient recipes for living to be very old and functioning well may have more relevance. For example, Hippocrates, the ancient Greek physician from nearly 3,000 years ago, simply believed that "everything in moderation" would lead to longevity. One thousand years later, his follower, the Roman physician Galen, prescribed "maintaining physical activity into old age, taking warm baths and massages regularly, and eating wisely especially fish, wine, figs, prunes, and honey" to live to a hundred. These methods are much closer to what current research suggests will extend life expectancy.

These days, we have carefully-researched longevity studies to help us determine what factors seem to explain why people live to be 100 years old and older—the "oldest old." Why do some people live to be 100 years of age while most do not? There are several scientific research projects in the U.S. that are studying the aging population and the rapidly-swelling group of people over 100 years of age. These major studies include the National Institutes of Mental Health Studies, the Baltimore Longitudinal Study of Aging the Framingham Heart and Aging Study, the Honolulu-Asia Heart and Aging Study, the Harvard Nurses and Health Professionals Studies, the California Seventh-Day Adventist Study, the MacArthur Successful Aging Study, the Georgia Centenarian Study, and the New

England Centenarian Study. Longevity and centenarian studies in Okinawa (including the famous Okinawan Centenarian Study), Japan (Chan et al, 1997); Italy (Capurso et al, 1997); Sweden (Samuelsson et al, 1997); France (Allard et al, 1994); Denmark (Jeune 1994); Hungary (Regius et al, 1994); the "Blue Zones" of Icaria (Greece), Costa Rica, and Sardinia (Buettner, 2008); and other countries are also producing valuable data on how and why certain people live to be 100 years and older.

From these two dozen or so longevity and centenarian studies, the body of information on the factors determining successful aging is accumulating rapidly. Although there are significant differences among individual centenarians, studies done in diverse parts of the world are finding some common factors that characterize groups of 100-year-olds. As noted by Dr. Perls of the New England Centenarian study, having a genetic advantage helps, but we can make lifestyle choices that increase the odds of achieving centenarian status. Centenarians make healthy lifestyle choices throughout their lives in order to live longer and healthier. Perls et al (1999) stated that, "One must stay healthy the vast majority of one's life in order to live to 100." Results from the existing centenarian studies around the world reveal similar healthy lifestyle characteristics. The secret is how to age well, not how to stay young.

THE "BLUE ZONES": WHERE DO PEOPLE LIVE THE LONGEST?

Where you live may make a difference, too. Dan Buettner, demographer and author of *The Blue Zones: Lessons for Living Longer from the People Who've Lived the Longest* (2008), has documented a number of areas of the world where there seem to be dense clusters of centenarians. He and his colleagues called these areas "Blue Zones," because of one researcher's habit of circling them on the map in blue ink. They include such diverse parts of the world as Okinawa; Sardinia; Costa Rica; and Loma Linda, California. Not surprisingly, most of the areas with high concentrations of centenarians have been physically and/or socially isolated from typical "western" cultural practices that negatively impact health and longevity.

The Japanese prefecture of Okinawa made up of hundreds of Ryukyu Islands stretching southward

Most of the areas with high concentrations of centenarians have been physically and/or socially isolated from typical "western" cultural practices that negatively impact health and longevity.

from the four main islands of Japan to the island of Taiwan. Okinawa Island, the largest in the chain, appears to have the population with the longest life expectancies and highest percentage of documented 100-year-olds in the world. Okinawans are mainly of peasant ancestry, racially distinct from mainland Japanese. Okinawan women live to 86 years and men to 78 years, which is significantly longer than mainland Japanese. There are an incredibly high number of centenarians and, amazingly, the vast majority of them are functionally independent. Okinawans live about seven years longer than Americans, have one-fifth the rate of heart disease, and have about four times as many people reach 100 years of age. The population has low rates of heart disease, diabetes, and dementia like Alzheimer's disease. They have excellent cardiovascular health, with low blood pressure, low blood cholesterol, and low levels of damaging free radicals. They also have low levels of hormone-dependent cancers and high bone densities with few fractures. Okinawans have youthful levels of sex hormones, including dihydroepiandrosterone (DHEA), estrogen, and testosterone—seemingly due to diets high in soy-based phytoestrogens, exercise, and other lifestyle factors. (No studies to date have demonstrated that taking these hormones or any other "anti-aging" supplements enhances the chances of reaching 100 years old.)

Overall, Okinawan centenarians tended to have the following common lifestyle practices:

1) having a purpose to life and a reason to get up each day, called an *ikigai*

2) eating a mostly plant-based diet with little meat that resembles the "Mediterranean Diet" for most of their lives

3) growing their own gardens, including medicinal gardens with healthy herbs

4) eating more soy

5) maintaining a stress-shedding social network called a *moai* and keeping younger people in their company

6) spend adequate time in sunlight to activate vitamin D

7) a high intake of calcium in the diet

8) staying active in activities like walking and gardening

9) having a high level of psychospiritual serenity

10) having high optimism and low levels of depression and anxiety disorders, and

11) having a strong but affable personality and attitude toward life and enjoying simple pleasures.

People who live in the internal, isolated, and mountainous Barbagia area of Sardinia have a very high likelihood of becoming centenarians. There are some atypical things about Sardinian centenarians. First of all, they are mostly men. This is in contrast the usual findings around the world where female centenarians outnumber male centenarians by about nine to one. The men are more active and live simpler lifestyles, while women are more sedentary and seem to have more stress in running their households.

These Sardinians in Barbagia also don't eat fish, which is somewhat unusual, but consume a lot of goat's milk and mastic oil.

As in other centenarians studies, lifestyle played the biggest role in achieving centenarian status. As noted by researcher Dr. Gianni Pes, "I suspect that the characteristics of the environment, the lifestyle, and the food are by far more important for a healthy life." Centenarians in the Barbagia region tended to have the following lifestyle practices:

1) eating a lean, plant-based diet with small amounts of red meat

2) having strong family connections and priorities with younger relatives closely involved with them

3) drinking goat's milk

4) celebrating and respecting their elders

5) walking several miles a day and working hard as farmers or shepherds most of their lives

6) drinking a glass or two of Cannanou red wine daily

7) having a lot of positive feelings, respect, and admiration for the elders of the society, and

8) lots of laughing and humor in their frequent social interactions with friends

The cluster of Seventh-Day Adventists living near Los Angeles in Loma Linda, California has been studied for several years. As noted in a July 9, 2001 *Archives of Internal Medicine* study, these Adventists outlive their fellow Californians by an average of nearly eight years and have a very high percentage of centenarians. California Seventh-Day Adventists tended to have the following lifestyle characteristics:

1) having a weekly stress-relieving break from life on the Sabbath to focus on family, camaraderie, and nature

2) possessing a high level of psychospiritual serenity

3) maintaining a low and healthy body weight

4) getting regular, moderate exercise

5) spending time with like-minded friends

6) snacking on nuts

7) finding purpose by volunteering and giving back to the community

8) following a mostly vegetarian diet with low levels of meat consumption

9) eating an early, light dinner

10) not smoking and not drinking alcohol, and

11) drinking five or six glasses of water per day

Compared to developed countries, the inhabitants of Costa Rica have very long life expectancies. The average Costa Rican man at age 60 years has twice the chance to reach age 90 years as a man in France, Japan, or the U.S. Although Costa Rica spends only 15 percent of what America does on health care, its people have longer, healthier lives. In particular, a group of villages around the isolated hills in the 80-mile-long Nicoya Peninsula bordering the Pacific Ocean may have the greatest percentage of centenarians in the country. Costa Rican centenarians in Nicoya tended to have the following lifestyle practices:

1) having a strong sense of purpose, called a *plan de vida*

2) wanting to contribute to the greater good of the community

3) drinking water with a high calcium and magnesium content

4) keeping a focus on the family

5) consuming fewer calories and eating a light dinner

6) consuming a largely vegetarian diet of corn, beans, garden vegetables, fruit, and some pork

7) maintaining social networks with lots of laughing and talking, and

8) keeping hard at work doing physical labor for most of their lives

In some smaller areas of the world, local populations may even outlive the Okinawans and have relatively more centenarians. One of these "Blue Zone" areas is the tiny Greek island of Icaria in the North Aegean Sea, which may have the highest concentration of people in the 90s and 100s in the world. Incredibly, about one in three inhabitants of this island make it into their 90s. Lifestyle plays a large role in this remarkable aging pattern. The island's inhabitants have an extremely low level of heart disease, cancers, depression, and dementia. They are physically active and walk a great deal, their diets are very high in olive oil, and they consume a wide variety of the 150 kinds of fruits and vegetables that grow wild on the island. They also drink herbal teas every day, morning and night. The fruits, vegetables, and herbal teas are all high in antioxidants, which apparently reduce free radical-induced aging. The teas are also diuretics, contributing to the Icarians' low blood pressure.

A cluster of Japanese-American men on the Hawaiian island of Oahu also have high numbers of centenarians. The Honolulu Aging Study has followed 8,000 Japanese-American men for many years. The study found that the oldest old of these men had low blood pressure and low blood sugar, did not smoke, and had body weights below the obesity level. The men who continued to follow a traditional Japanese diet and lifestyle had the highest chance of making it to 100 years of age. The Japanese Centenarian Study found similar predictors.

Unfortunately, as noted by Buettner (2008), the people who make it to very, very old age in these areas are starting to disappear. This is due to the encroachment of industrialized culture by fast food, television, and "labor-saving" technology. Younger people and even older people in their 50s, 60s, and 70s are now tending to eat more "junk" processed foods, be overweight, ride in cars and trucks instead of walking and exercising, watch television, and having more stress than their centenarian counterparts. Even in Okinawa, longevity may soon become a province of women only. According to Buettner (2008), Hormel exports approximately five million pounds of Spam a year to Okinawa, and Okinawans now eat more hamburgers per capita than any of Japan's other 47 prefectures. Okinawan men are now among the most obese in all of Japan and do not live much longer than the average Japanese man. In these high-longevity "Blue Zone" areas of the world, adopting a more "western" lifestyle may mean that the high numbers of centenarians may soon be a thing of the past.

CENTENARIANS: WHAT THEY HAVE IN COMMON AROUND THE WORLD

Centenarians seem to share several common lifestyle characteristics no matter where they live in the world. In reviewing several centenarian studies, Flanigan and Sawyer (2007) found 10 such commonalities among the oldest, healthiest people in the world:

1) low cholesterol

2) low blood pressure

3) non-smoking

4) diets rich in fish, fruit, and vegetables

5) regular exercise

6) healthy weight

7) avoiding accidents

8) low alcohol intake

9) taking low-dose aspirin, and

10) taking a multivitamin

In "Blue Zones," Buettner (2008) found nine characteristics that the concentrations of centenarians from Okinawa, Sardinia, Costa Rica, and Loma Linda, California seemed to share:

1) staying active with daily physical exercise

2) eating fewer calories

3) eating mostly fruits and vegetables with low amounts of meat and processed foods

4) drinking red wine in moderation

5) having a purpose and a clear goal in life

6) taking time to reduce stress

7) participating in a spiritual community

8) making family a priority and putting loved ones first, and

9) being surrounded by people who shared similar healthy lifestyle values

One particular group of centenarians that are of particular interest is those who have maintained the ability to live on their own. Amazingly, 20 to 30 percent of centenarians still live independently, and another

20 percent have the capacity to do so even though they live with other people. These vigorous people seem to have remarkably intact cognitive, physical, and emotional status with minimal levels of frailty at this highly advanced age. Some studies, such as the Georgia Centenarian Study and Japanese Centenarian Study, have researched this group extensively.

The Georgia study found independently-living centenarians to have the following characteristics:

1) no smoking history

2) normal weight without large weight fluctuations

3) very little alcohol consumption

4) very physically active throughout life

5) eat breakfast on a daily basis

6) avoid weight loss diets

7) good everyday cognitive problem-solving and coping skills

8) higher education

9) a relaxed, practical, non-stressful personality style

10) a good family and friend support system

11) have no clinical depression or other significant emotional symptoms, and

12) generally practice good health habits that prolong life (Poon et al, 1992)

In the Japanese Centenarian Study, independent living 100-year-olds were associated with:

1) better visual acuity

2) regular exercise

3) spontaneous morning awakening

4) preserved masticatory ability

5) no history of drinking alcohol

6) no history of severe falls after age 95 years

7) more frequent intake of protein, and

8) being male (even though there are more women centenarians, men are much more likely to live independently)

How to Live to 100 Years Old: The 16 Steps

By examining all the available aging studies, certain common features of the most functional centenarians start to emerge. Successful aging is typically found in people with a cluster of lifestyle characteristics and genes associated with a long and healthy life, not just one or two things. In particular, independent-living centenarians—possibly the role models for slowing the aging process—are often found to be remarkably similar in several aspects of their lives no matter where in the world they live. When it comes to those lifestyle predictors associated with people who have the longest, healthiest, and most cognitively intact lifespans, the whole seems to be greater than the sum of its parts. Want to live to be 100 and

> **Successful aging is typically found in people with a cluster of lifestyle characteristics and genes associated with a long and healthy life, not just one or two things.**

still be healthy and doing well? An analysis of the two dozen existing centenarian and human aging studies suggest that you might try following all or even a cluster of some of these 16 steps that represent lifestyle characteristics commonly shared by centenarians around the world:

Step 1: Maintain Low Blood Sugar

Cardiovascular disease is the major killer of Americans, and high blood sugar (glucose) in the form of diabetes is a major risk for developing it. While more than half of today's 74 million "baby boomers" will live past age 85 years, most of them will succumb to chronic diseases like heart disease, stroke, and diabetes before reaching 100 unless they take steps to avoid risk factors. Since cardiovascular risk factors contribute to early death rates, it is not surprising that those factors are far less prevalent in centenarians when compared to younger old individuals (Galioto et al, 2008).

Centenarians tend to have low blood sugar compared to the average American—usually a fasting blood sugar below 100. This low level of blood sugar has been found in centenarian studies around the world (Zyczkowska et al, 2006), including the Honolulu Heart/Aging Study. C.J. Murray and colleagues (Murray, Kulkami, & Ezzati, 2005) found in their study of American life expectancies that low blood sugar was a major factor in predicting a long and healthy life.

Many physicians and scientists who

> **High blood sugar and diabetes may represent the model for accelerated aging and a shortened lifespan.**

study successful and healthy aging, such as Andrew Weil, MD., believe that high blood sugar and diabetes may represent the model for accelerated aging and a shortened lifespan. Chronic high blood sugar in the form of insulin resistance and diabetes damage the body in numerous ways. Diabetes is the fifth leading cause of death in the U. S. and, if present, powerfully reduces the chance of living to 100 years of age. Studies have found that diabetes mellitus in supercentenarians over 110 years of age is rare (Schoenhofen et al, 2006).

Unfortunately, high blood sugar is becoming a worldwide public health problem, particularly in industrialized nations. Prediabetes, a condition found in 57 million Americans, is characterized by a fasting glucose level of 100 to 125 mg/dL, or an oral glucose tolerance test of 140 to 200 mg/dL. Diabetes results when glucose levels exceed those ranges. One type of diabetes, *type 1* or *juvenile-onset diabetes*, is genetic. The other major type, *type 2* or *adult-onset diabetes*, is due to lifestyle habits and is typically brought on by obesity, high-calorie and high-fat diets, and lack of exercise. It is type 2 diabetes that is becoming a worldwide pandemic in industrialized countries.

The new target fasting blood glucose level recommended by the American Diabetes Association (ADA) and the American College of Endocrinology (ACE) is a fasting glucose below 100 mg/dL and an oral glucose tolerance test below 140 mg/dL. Centenarians typically have blood sugar around or under these levels. Having blood glucose above these levels raises the risk for coronary heart disease, stroke, foot and skin infections, and kidney, eye, and nerve damage. Both high and low blood sugar levels are a problem in diabetes. If glucose levels are chronically high (*hyperglycemia*), the chances of these life-shortening diseases increases. The *hypoglycemic* episodes (very low blood sugar) common in diabetics have recently been linked in an increased risk for Alzheimer's disease. Keeping blood sugar or glucose low is an open secret to healthy aging and is an important first step in reaching 100 years old.

Step 2: Maintain Low Blood Pressure

As noted earlier, a key to making it to 100 years old is to avoid cardiovascular disease. Very few centenarians in the New England Centenarian Study were found to have long-term histories of heart disease. A large number of studies have demonstrated that centenarians and supercentenarians (110 years and older) have better cardiovascular risk profiles compared to typical younger old people in their 70s, 80s, and 90s (Galioto et al, 2008; Schoenhofen et al, 2006). In particular, centenarian studies around the world have consistently found lower blood pressures in 100-year-olds compared to the average levels of younger 70- and 80-year-olds (Samuelsson et al, 1997). Examination of centenarians in the New England Centenarian Study generally revealed systolic blood pressures no higher

Centenarians and supercentenarians *(110 years and older)* have better cardiovascular risk profiles compared to typical younger old people in their 70s, 80s, and 90s.

than 110 and diastolic pressures lower than 80. The inhabitants of Icaria, have remarkably low blood pressure. Diabetes, angina, and myocardial infarction (heart attack) are also typically less common in centenarians than in 70- and 80-year-olds (Zyczkowska et al, 2006), and hypertension is an independent risk factor for all these diseases.

Blood pressure is the force of blood pushing against the walls of the arteries, and is the result of two different forces. *Systolic blood pressure* (the first, higher number) is generated when the heart's lower chambers, the ventricles, "beat" by contracting and pushing blood into the arteries of the circulatory system. At rest, the heart commonly beats about 60 to 70 times a minute. *Diastolic blood pressure* (the second, lower number) is created by the arteries' resistance to blood flow between heartbeats. Blood pressure usually increases with physical activity, nervousness, and excitement. Even the time of day can make a difference as pressure is lowest during sleep and rises when awakening. Many things can increase blood pressure, including obesity, smoking, lack of exercise, certain hormones, stress, atherosclerosis, the amount of water in the bloodstream, and sodium.

Sodium is an essential nutrient that is usually consumed as dietary salt or sodium chloride. Sodium intake regulates fluid balances in the bloodstream and body. High sodium levels in the body are associated with increased water retention and higher blood pressure. Adults need about 400 to 500 mg of sodium per day for optimal nutrition—about one-fourth of a teaspoon of salt. It recommended daily consumption should not exceed 1,500 mg. Unfortunately, many Americans eat up to 4,000 mg of sodium a day, much of which comes not from a salt shaker but from the added salt in processed foods. A high intake of sodium is directly related to high blood pressure, which affects about one-third of Americans and is a powerful risk factor for heart disease and stroke. Cutting salt intake and increasing potassium intake is a good way to help lower blood pressure.

Hypertension is defined as a blood pressure greater than 140 millimeters of mercury (mmHg) systolic and 90 mmHg diastolic. When blood flows through arteries

Table 3. *Levels of Blood Pressure*

Category	Blood Pressure
Normal	Less than 120/80
Prehypertension	120/80 to 139/89
Isolated Systolic Hypertension	Over 140/Less than 90
Stage 1 Hypertension*	140/90 to 159/99
Stage 2 Hypertension	160 or higher/100 or higher

An exception would be in persons with diabetes and/or chronic kidney disease, where 130/80 is considered hypertension.

at high pressure for a long time, it damages the inner layer of the arteries (the *endothelium*). This opens the door for the development of atherosclerotic plaque and heart disease. Hypertension damages not only the arteries of the heart and brain, causing heart attacks and stroke, but also injures blood vessels throughout the body, which can lead to limb amputation, kidney disease, and blindness. Although the exact cause of hypertension remains elusive in most cases, it is clear how blood pressure can be lowered and controlled in most cases. If you don't keep it under control, you are at very high risk for heart disease and stroke. Until age 55, more American men have hypertension than women. After age 55, more women develop hypertension.

Unfortunately, hypertension is very likely to happen in most older Americans. Of those in the U.S. with normal blood pressure in the 50s, 90 percent will eventually develop hypertension if they live into their 80s. The type of hypertension that will occur in 90 percent of older Americans is isolated systolic hypertension, where the systolic goes over 140 mmHg and the diastolic stays under 90. However, this type of hypertension is no walk in the park. The Framingham Heart Study has found that high systolic blood pressure is far more predictive of who will develop heart disease and require treatment than high diastolic pressure.

The new target blood pressure for optimal heart health according to the American Heart Association (AHA) is under 120/80, at 115/75. Why is this important? Because a 2002 meta-analysis of 61 different studies of one million adults found that, above 115/75, every 20-point increase over a systolic blood pressure of 115 and every 10-point increase above a diastolic pressure of 75 doubles the risk of heart attack. When blood pressure increases from 115/75 to 135/85, the risk for heart attacks doubles; when it increases from 115/75 to 155/95, the risk quadruples. And, when blood pressure increases from 115/75 to 175/105, the risk of a heart attack is eight times as great and the risk of a stroke increases 12-fold!

Even small increases in blood pressure can be dangerous to health. For example, the Framingham Heart Study found that even high-normal blood pressure of 130 to 139 over 85 to 89 increased a woman's chance of developing cardiovascular disease by 60 percent and a man's chance by a whopping 150 percent over a 10-year period compared to those with normal blood pressure.

High blood pressure also damages the brain. Honolulu Aging Study researchers found that for every increase of 10 mg/Hg in systolic blood pressure in midlife, there was a seven to nine percent increase in the risk for impaired cognitive function. So, it is critical to control blood pressure and keep it relatively low if you want a long and healthy life. The bad news is that the average American blood pressure is about 130/80—well above where it should be for optimal health and longevity.

Diet, lifestyle, and anti-hypertensive drugs can work to keep blood pressure at the target levels of 115 mmHg systolic and 75 mmHg diastolic or below. Centenarians typically have diets that resemble the Mediterranean and Dietary Approaches to Stop Hypertension (DASH) diets, which are associated with low blood pressure. The "Blue Zone" Icarians drink herbal tea on a daily basis that is a diuretic, helping lower their blood pressure. The oldest old typically have lifestyles associated with low blood pressure that include frequent exercise, low stress, low alcohol intake, and not smoking. Because of their diets and lifestyle, centenarians have been found to take lower levels of anti-hypertensive drugs at younger ages, i.e., in their 70s, 80s, and 90s, than non-centenarians. However, if diet and exercise don't work, lowering blood pressure by taking anti-hypertensive medications may play an important role in reaching the oldest ages. Some studies have shown that as many as 20 percent of supercentenarians over 110 years of age are taking medications for hypertension (Schoenhofen et al, 2006). Annual physical examinations including testing for blood pressure are important for identifying any elevations that should be addressed and lowered. If your blood pressure is elevated, implement lifestyle changes or take antihypertensive medications to keep blood pressure low.

Step 3: Have Low Blood Total Cholesterol

You are not likely to live a long time if your arteries are stiff and clogged with cholesterol-laden atherosclerotic plaque. *Cholesterol* is a waxy, fatlike substance mostly produced in the liver that is an essential ingredient in hormones and cellular structures. About one gram per day is produced by the liver and is all that most people need, but many Americans absorb another superfluous half gram a day from the consumption of dietary egg yolks, meat, fish, poultry, and whole-milk dairy products. This excess cholesterol can find its way into the artery walls as deposits that develop into artery-stiffening and clot-producing atherosclerotic plaque. A major obstacle to achieving centenarian status is the development of atherosclerotic plaque in the arteries. This plaque, along with hypertension, is the major cause of heart disease and stroke. As noted earlier, heart disease and stroke kill about as many Americans as the next five leading causes of death together, including cancer. Heart disease and stroke comprise cardiovascular disease, a disorder largely resulting from the build-up of plaque in the arteries that disrupts the supply of oxygenated blood to the heart and brain. This plaque can rupture, causing the clots that result in heart attacks and strokes. Many centenarians markedly delay the clinical expression of cardiovascular disease until the very end of their exceptionally long lives or avoid the disease entirely (Schoenhofen et al, 2006).

You are not likely to live a long time if your arteries are stiff and clogged with cholesterol-laden atherosclerotic plaque.

Two kinds of fats are found in blood serum, *cholesterol* and *triglycerides*. From these two fats, there are four scores measured by a fasting blood test. One is the amount of triglycerides in the blood. Excess calories are converted into triglycerides and transported to fat cells for storage as energy. Triglyercides are composed of three fatty acids held together by glycerol. Triglyceride levels less than 150 mg/dL are optimal, and levels over 200 are high and a risk for cardiovascular disease.

There are two main types of cholesterol. *Low-density lipoproteins (LDL)*, called "bad" cholesterol, are combination fat-protein molecules that carry cholesterol from the liver into the bloodstream. The optimal level of LDL is less than 100 mg/dL. LDL levels over 160 mg/dL pose a cardiovascular disease risk. *High-density lipoproteins (HDL)*, called "good" cholesterol, are fat-protein molecules that carry cholesterol out of the bloodstream and back to the liver. Total cholesterol is determined by adding (1) the LDL level, (2) the HDL level, and (3) one-fifth of the triglyceride level. Total cholesterol should optimally be less than 200 mg/dL. Over 240 mg/dL total cholesterol is considered to be high and a risk for cardiovascular disease.

The levels of blood fats—especially cholesterol— have a tremendous impact on the development of atherosclerotic plaque and subsequent cardiovascular disease. Atherosclerosis begins with damage to the inner layer of arteries. This damage can come from high blood pressure or tobacco toxins, high blood sugar, or inflammation. About 70 percent of body cholesterol is transported by LDL cholesterol.

The damaged endothelium lets LDL cholesterol into the inner part of the artery, called the intima, where cholesterol begins to be deposited. The damaged endothelial cells and cholesterol build-up attracts white blood cells to repair the damage, causing inflammation in the arteries. The white blood cells begin engulfing the cholesterol and become large foam cells. The free radicals secreted by these cells oxidize elements in the plaque, including cholesterol, making it larger and creating scar tissue. As the plaque enlarges, it is filled with large foam cells, cholesterol, smooth muscle cells, platelets, and scar tissue. When the foam cells finally die, their fatty contents are released into the plaque, forming a liquid necrotic core. A cap composed of cells and clots is then formed over the plaque to hold it in. This cap later hardens with deposits of calcium. If this cap ruptures, which it often does, the plaque material spills into the bloodstream, causing the formation of a clot. If this clot occurs in the drinking-straw sized arteries of the heart or in the arteries of the brain, a heart attack or stroke will result. High blood total cholesterol, high LDL cholesterol, low HDL cholesterol, and high triglycerides can all contribute to the development of atherosclerotic plaque.

As might be expected, those people who make it to 100 years old, on the whole, have impressively young and clean arteries with low LDL cholesterol and low total cholesterol compared to elderly individuals in their 70s and 80s in the normal population (Zyczkowska et al, 2006). Some centenarians studied at autopsy have had arteries that were virtually free of atherosclerotic plaque (Berstein, Willcox, et al, 2004). Centenarians also have lower blood levels of fibrinogen, which converts to fibrin, the fibrous protein that holds platelets together and forms blood clots. A low level of serum homocysteine, an amino acid that damages arterial walls, is also found in Okinawan centenarians. If your arteries are flexible, resilient, and free of cholesterol-laden plaque, many years will probably be added to your life.

Keeping blood total cholesterol levels low cannot be emphasized enough. Dr. William Castelli, a former lead researcher of the Framingham Heart Study, has stated that, "In forty years, we never found a heart attack in anyone with cholesterol below 150…Close to 90 percent of all coronary death could be prevented if the cholesterol was kept below 182 mg/dL, blood pressure under 120 mmHg, and no smoking or diabetes" (Flanigan & Sawyer, 2007, p. 37). As noted by Dr. William Roberts, editor of *The American Journal of Cardiology*, "the only *absolute* prerequisite for a fatal or nonfatal atherosclerotic event is a serum total cholesterol level greater than 150 mg/dL." (Flanigan and Sawyer, 2007). Heart disease and stroke are largely preventable diseases. Keeping the four key blood lipids within healthy ranges helps keep the arteries free of plaque and plays a major role in a long and healthy life. The target levels of the three major cholesterols and triglycerides are:

- *Total Cholesterol:* under 200 mg/dL; optimally under 150 mg/dL

- *LDL Cholesterol:* under 100 mg/dL; optimally under 70 mg/dL

- *HDL Cholesterol:* more than 45 mg/dL; optimally more than 50 mg/dL

- *Triglycerides:* under 150 mg/dL; optimally under 100 mg/dL

- *Total Cholesterol/HDL Ratio:* less than 3.5; optimally less than 3.0

It is important to realize that lifestyle, not genetics, has the greatest impact on total cholesterol levels in most of us. A study that followed middle-aged Japanese immigrants from Japan to Hawaii to California illustrates this dramatically. The men living in Japan had an average total cholesterol of 140 mg/dL, but the average level of total cholesterol in the Hawaiian immigrants was 200 mg/dL. When they moved to the Los Angeles area, the average total cholesterol shot up to 150 mg/dL. The American diet and lifestyle caused this dramatic increase, not genetics.

The good news is that building atherosclerotic plaque usually takes decades, and is preventable and even reversible with lifestyle changes and medications. The AHA recommends consuming less than 300 mg of dietary cholesterol per day (one egg yolk contains 300 mg of cholesterol) to help keep blood levels low. Saturated fats and transfatty acids (trans fats) also markedly increase serum cholesterol and LDL cholesterol. Dr. Michael Clearfield of North Texas State University noted that if the average American's LDL cholesterol was kept below 100 mg/dL, heart disease would disappear as a major cause of death. When LDL cholesterol is lowered below 100, plaque volume reduces. Regular physical activity, eating a healthy diet, keeping weight below the overweight level, and avoiding or stopping smoking are ways to reduce LDL cholesterol. Also, statin drugs can reduce LDL cholesterol, total cholesterol, triglycerides, and inflammation enough to lower heart disease risk by 30 percent. Exercise, diet, fibrates, and niacin can all raise HDL cholesterol and possibly lower triglycerides. The omega-3 polyunsaturated fatty acids in fish oil can also lower cholesterol and triglycerides. For some people, especially men, daily low-dose aspirin therapy may reduce the chances of blood clots, and have a significant effect on life extension and the chances of reaching 100 years of age.

Step 4: Keep Weight Low and Steady

One characteristic of all the aging studies is that people who live to the oldest age and remain healthy have low body weights, presumably due to low caloric diet and regular exercise. Centenarians are almost always lean and fit, and most have never been obese. In the New England Centenarian Study, 99 percent of the participants did not meet the criteria for obesity. This is important, because obesity, along with smoking, is the biggest killer of Americans and a major cause of shortened life expectancy. Obesity leads to inefficient energy production in the body and an increased production of oxygen-free radicals within cells, leading to accelerated aging. Being obese or overweight is a major risk factor for more than 30 serious medical conditions, including heart disease; stroke; hypertension; type 2 diabetes; Alzheimer's disease; and many forms of cancer, including colon, rectal, and prostate cancer in men and gallbladder, breast, cervix, uterine, and ovarian cancer in women. A 13-year American Cancer Society study found that both men and women whose body weight was 40 percent greater than average for their height and age group had dramatically greater risks for cancer than those with normal weights—33 percent greater for men and 35 percent greater for women.

> **People who live to the oldest age and remain healthy have low body weights.**

Centenarians typically have gained little or no weight during their adult years. In the New England Centenarian Study, 80 percent of participants said their weight was close to what they weighed for their entire adult lives. Okinawan centenarians, for example, have an average BMI that ranged from 18 to 22 (normal range is 18.5 to 24.9). The average American BMI exceeds 26, since nearly two-thirds of Americans are overweight or obese. Waist circumference or the waist-hip ratio is also an important measure of obesity, since abdominal visceral fat under the muscles and next to the organs is a particularly dangerous risk for the development of cardiovascular disease and diabetes. If a man's waist exceeds 40 inches or a woman's exceeds 35 inches, this presents a dangerous threat to health even if the BMI is in the normal range. Centenarians typically have narrow waists with a small amount of visceral abdominal fat.

Being a lacto-ovo vegetarian (one who eats eggs and other dairy products) or a vegan is strongly associated with low body weights. In the Seventh-Day Adventist Health Study, lacto-ovo vegetarians were an average of 16 pounds lighter than individuals of the same height who were not vegetarians. Adventists who were strictly vegan (only four percent), were a whopping 30 to 32 pounds lighter than non-vegetarians of the same height.

The dramatic increase in obesity in the United States and other developed countries over the last few decades is startling and may play a role in reducing the number of future centenarians. Obesity now accounts for 300,000 deaths per year in the U.S., about equal to deaths caused by smoking. In the last 20 years, the obesity rates in American adults and children have doubled, while the rate of adolescent obesity has tripled! In 2003 to 2006 data, the CDC found 34 percent of American adults to be obese and 30 percent to be overweight. In recent years, women have gained more weight than men. There are sex and ethnic differences in obesity in the U.S. Among those Americans between the ages of 40 to 59, the obesity rate is 40 percent among all men but 51 percent of Mexican-American women and 53 percent of African-American women are now obese. Above the age of 60 years, 61 percent of African-American women are obese. Child obesity is also becoming a huge problem in the U.S. A recent study by Anderson and Whitaker in the *Archives of Pediatrics and Adolescent Medicine* found that a surprising 18 percent of four-year-olds in the U.S. were already obese. These high levels have never been seen before in the U.S.

If someone is overweight or obese, losing weight is critical to health and longevity. Beginning any of the myriad of advertised diets is not usually very effective, as only about five percent of people will lose weight on these diets and keep it off for at least two years. Among the low-fat, low-carbohydrate, and high-protein diets that are widely marketed, two-year follow-up studies show no significant difference in weight loss These commonly-advertised diets are all basically low-calorie diets in disguise and are difficult to stay on for long periods of time, often because they are boring and the food isn't tasty enough.

What diet is most effective over time? It is the same as the diet that appears to be the healthiest—the "Mediterranean diet" *(see Step 6).* A major July, 2008 study in the *New England Journal of Medicine* found that this diet resulted in more long-term weight loss and better glycemic control than low-carbohydrate or low-fat diets. It is healthier than a low-carbohydrate diet and easier to follow than a low-fat diet. The Mediterranean diet is naturally low in "bad" saturated and trans fats and high in taste, which makes it a good choice for the major long-term lifestyle changes necessary for life-long weight control. Eating small portions, keeping calories down, and making changes in lifestyle choices are also important in using this diet for weight loss.

Losing weight and keeping it off requires a planned and disciplined lifestyle change. To look at how people have successfully lost an average of 66 pounds and kept it off for over five years, take a look at the people in the National Weight Control Registry associated with

Brown Medical School at *www.nwcr.ws*. The Registry, established in 1994 by Rena Wing, PhD and James Hill, PhD, provides stark evidence that people lose weight and keep it off for long periods of time using diverse methods. About half of the 5,000 people in the Registry who lost weight and kept it off did it on their own, while the other half did it with the help of a formal program. Although Registry participants lost weight in a variety of ways, the data show that people who sustained their weight loss tended to do a number of similar things:

- 78 percent eat breakfast every day

- 75 percent weigh themselves at least once a week

- 62 percent watch less than 10 hours of television per week, and

- 90 percent exercise, on average, about one hour per day.

As might be expected, these were also found to be the habits of independent-living centenarians with normal weights in the Georgia Centenarian Study.

Keeping weight in the average range appears to be a prerequisite for achieving centenarian status.

Step 5: Eat Fewer Calories

What is the one thing that has been found to extend the lifespan of several animal species? Eating fewer calories. Caloric restriction with optimal nutrition significantly lowers heart disease, stroke, diabetes, and cancer risk factors and extends life spans as much as genetic manipulation (Walford and Walford, 2005; Willcox et al, 2006). In an age when the average American eats 2,500 to 3,000 calories per day, those who eat closer to 1,800 to 2,000 calories per day with adequate nutrition levels live much longer—and are much more likely to live beyond 100 years.

As the body ages after age 20 years, 100 fewer calories per day are required during each additional decade. If 2,500 calories per day were eaten by someone with a normal weight at age 20 years, that person will require only 2,000 calories by age 70 years and 1,700 by age 100 years. The famous "middle-age spread" results from people continuing to eat at the same level as they age. The excess calories not required to run the body functions are stored as fat.

Centenarian studies commonly find that the oldest old often consume a relatively

> **Caloric restriction with optimal nutrition significantly lowers heart disease, stroke, diabetes, and cancer risk factors and extends life spans.**

low number of calories per day. Okinawans eat about 20 percent fewer calories per day than Americans, and live nearly six years longer on average (84 years to 78 years). Japanese researchers found that Okinawans consumed 17 percent fewer calories than mainland Japanese, and had 31 to 41 percent lower death rates from heart disease, stroke, and cancer. Okinawans practice a Confucian-based cultural way of eating called *hara hachi bu,* which means eating until they are about 80 percent full and then ceasing eating before they reach satiation. According to Craig Willcox, "Okinawa may be the only human population that purposefully restricts how many calories they eat and they do it by reminding themselves to eat until they're 80 percent full." (Buetter, 2008). Not only that, centenarians typically will eat meals that contain mostly foods with low caloric density like fruits and vegetables. Such a meal can have a volume of four times that of a hamburger but contain only one-half the calories. So, stopping before feeling full means even fewer calories are consumed. Even with active lifestyles, centenarians across all studies typically eat less than 2,000 calories per day, and often much less than that.

Eating fewer calories appears to slow down the body's metabolic rate and reduce the production of mitochrondrial free radicals that cumulatively damage vital body molecules over time and lead to early death. Okinawans following their traditional lifestyle have been shown to have low blood levels of free radicals and less free-radical damage to their bodies.

The cardiovascular benefits of caloric restriction are nothing less than astounding. A study in the Netherlands found that men who reduced their caloric intake by 20 percent for 10 weeks had increased HDL levels, reduced blood pressure, and a achieved a 10 percent loss in body weight. In a study in the 2004 *Proceedings of the National Academy of Science*, Luigi Fontana and colleagues at Washington University in St. Louis studied caloric restriction in volunteers over three years and, compared to those on regular American diets, those who ate about 20 to 25 percent fewer calories less per day lowered total cholesterol from 204 to 170, lowered LDL cholesterol from 123 to 86, raised HDL cholesterol, lowered triglycerides from 150 to 56, and lowered blood pressure from 130/80 to 100/60. Directly relevant to successful aging, eating fewer calories has also been shown to increase life span in several studies (Heilbronn LK et al, 2003; Sohal et al, 1996). Clearly, caloric restriction with optimal nutrition is part of the path to the century mark.

Step 6: Eat a Mostly Vegetarian "Mediterranean" Diet with Coffee/Tea

It's an old maxim: We are what we eat. And, basically, we are vegetarians. Humans are technically omnivores; that is, we are able to eat and digest both meat and plants. However, our bodies are really designed to eat plants. We are basically herbivores like cows and gorillas, not carnivores like dogs and cats. We have flat molars for grinding, no claws, weak stomach acids, and very long intestinal tracts for nutrient absorption—all designed for eating plants, not meat. Centenarians across all studies have a diet mostly made up of plant-based foods like fruits, vegetables, roots, beans and peas, nuts, and grains. For example, in the MEDIS study of elderly people living on Mediterranean islands, the longest-lived had a strong adherence to the "Mediterranean" diet (Tourlouki et al, 2009).

> **Centenarians across all studies have a diet mostly made up of plant-based foods.**

One of the big differences between carnivores and herbivores is that carnivores don't develop atherosclerotic plaque in their arteries, but herbivores do. Since we are basically designed to be herbivores, we get atherosclerosis. However, eating meat, while a good source of protein, zinc, and iron, can help cause arterial plaque when eaten in large quantities. Across all studies, centenarians typically eat a largely plant-based diet and eat red meat only occasionally.

The most commonly-seen dietary pattern in centenarians resembles what has come to be called the Mediterranean diet. Beginning with studies in the 1960s in Crete and later with the 1980s "Seven Countries Study," research has found that a diet resembling that of countries that border the Mediterranean Sea appears to be associated with longer and healthier lives. Basically, the Mediterranean diet is:

1) high in calories from whole grains, fruits, and vegetables

2) medium in calories from nuts, beans, peas, fish, poultry, and eggs, and

3) low in calories from saturated fat dairy products, red meat, and refined carbohydrates (table sugar, refined flour, white potatoes, white rice, and some pastas).

The Mediterranean diet also has a relatively high level of monosaturated and polyunsaturated fats found in olive oil, canola oil, nuts, and avocados. A major review in the September, 2008 *British Medical Journal* found that the Mediterranean diet was associated with the longest life expectancies of any diet because it was associated with the fewest deaths from cardiovascular disease, cancer, Parkinson's disease, and Alzheimer's disease. Many studies, including the Harvard nutrition and aging studies, show that individuals living the longest and staying the healthiest get their highest number of calories from a diet of whole grains, plant fats and oils, fruits, vegetables, nuts, beans, and peas that resembles the Mediterranean diet (Willett, 2001). Eating this kind of diet benefits healthy aging in a number of ways. For example, studies of Okinawan centenarians show that the isoflavones absorbed from eating soybeans regularly apparently slow bone loss and ease menopausal hot flashes (Messina et al, 2004; Albertazzi et al, 1998). The Adventist Health Study found that eating nuts regularly added two years to life expectancy. Among all the choices available, the Mediterranean diet is probably the best in the world for healthy aging.

> **A diet resembling that of countries that border the Mediterranean Sea appears to be associated with longer and healthier lives.**

Centenarians typically consume small amounts of red meat, saturated fat from dairy products, trans fats from fried and baked foods, and refined carbohydrates. Death from heart disease—the biggest threat to life—is strongly related to intake of saturated fats and trans fats in these foods. We've known this since World War II when it was found that heart disease rates in Norway and Finland significantly declined during the German occupation. During that time, many of the foods high in saturated fat such as red meat and dairy products were in short supply. When the war was over and these foods were again being consumed in large quantities, the number of deaths from heart attacks soared.

Eating red meat has been shown to be associated with heart disease, cancers, and a shortened life span in numerous studies. The Adventist Health Study found that those who ate red meat had twice the risk of heart disease compared to vegetarians. This study also found that red meat eaters had significantly more cancers compared to vegetarians, including a 65 percent higher risk for colon and ovarian cancers. One less serving of meat each day would reduce the number of colon cancer cases by 11 percent (Perls et al, 1999). A vegetarian Seventh-Day Adventist typically lived two years longer than those who ate meat. A 2009 study of 500,000 people followed by the National Cancer Institute showed that men and women who ate a lot of red meat and processed meats such as hot dogs and bacon were more than 30 percent more likely to die during a 10-year period than people who rarely consumed these foods. As noted by epidemiologist Barry Popkin, "You eat a hot dog a week and you're going to up, quite a bit, your risk of death in a 10-year period." The culprits are thought to be the saturated fat in red meat and the carcinogens from it, along with the added salt and carcinogenic nitrites in processed meats. In addition, cooking meat until it is charred adds cancer risk from the damaging heterocyclic amines that are formed. Nearly all the centenarians around the world in the various studies have consumed red meat only occasionally, if at all.

The refined carbohydrates that form such a large part of the American diet pose a particular danger to health because of their association with high blood sugar and the risks of insulin resistance and diabetes. The famed heart surgeon Michael DeBakey once remarked that, "Anything white will kill you." Those "white" foods he warned about were refined carbohydrates with high glycemic indexes such as table sugar, high-fructose corn syrup, white flour, white potatoes, white rice, and white pasta. As noted earlier, 30 percent of calories consumed daily by the average American come from a combination of (1) alcohol and (2) sugar or high fructose corn syrup. Bread was shown in a recent study in the *American Journal of Clinical Nutrition* to be the food contributing the most calories to enlarged waist sizes and overall obesity in Americans. Centenarians typically consume low amounts of these foods and additives.

In particular, the Mediterranean diet is characterized by a large intake of a variety of fruits and vegetables— resembling the way our Stone Age ancestors ate. Numerous studies have shown that eating lots of fruits and vegetables extends life expectancy and lowers the risk of many age-related diseases such as colon, lung, and prostate cancers; cardiovascular disease; vision problems; rheumatoid arthritis; diabetes; Parkinson's disease; and Alzheimer's disease (Perls et al, 1999). Harvard researchers estimate that if all Americans ate the recommended five servings of fruits and vegetables each day, there would be a 20 percent decrease in lung cancer and an increase in life expectancies.

For example, Seventh-Day Adventists are largely vegetarians and have a very high percentage of centenarians. The Adventist Health Study found that a 30-year-old vegetarian Seventh-Day Adventist man will live 9.5 years longer than the average 30-year-old California man. An Adventist vegetarian woman lives 6.1 years longer than the average California woman after age 30 years. Eating "colorful" fruits and vegetables helps supply a wide variety of micronutrients, especially plant antioxidants that blunt the free-radical damage that accelerates aging of the body and brain. The leading neuroscientist James Joseph at Tufts University has documented the cognitive benefits from the antioxidants in blueberries in numerous studies. "There are over 200 different carotenoids and 200 different flavonoids in a single tomato," says Luigi Ferrucci of the Baltimore aging study, "and these chemicals can all have complex interactions that foster health beyond the single nutrients we know about, like lycopene or vitamin C."

Eating fruits and vegetables adds antioxidants to the body and also seems to promote the production of the body's own antioxidants. Studies have shown that centenarians have significantly higher amounts of internally-produced antioxidants such as glutathione reductase and glutathione catalase than are found in young healthy adults (Klapcinska et al, 2000). In general, the more fruits and vegetables consumed on a daily basis, the longer the life expectancy. Okinawans—the longest-lived in the world with the highest percentage of centenarians—eat seven servings of fruits and vegetables per day compared to just over two for the average American. Probably because of eating lots of green leafy green vegetables and having a high intake of vitamins B_6 and B_{12}, Okinawan centenarians also have low levels of a damaging amino acid called homocysteine, high levels of which are associated with arterial wall damage and Alzheimer's disease. To give you an idea of how important a mostly vegetarian diet is, when native Okinawans move to Western countries—and adopt a more Western-style diet—they lose several years of their life expectancy.

Are there any "superfoods" in a mostly vegetarian diet that have an especially strong impact on health and longevity? According to the December 2003 *Nutrition Action Health Letter*, the top 10 superfoods to include in a healthy diet are sweet potatoes (eaten often by Okinawans); grape tomatoes; fat-free or one percent milk; broccoli; salmon; whole grain crackers; brown rice; citrus fruits; butternut squash; and numerous greens, including kale and spinach. Foods also consumed in abundance by centenarians include nuts, blueberries, olive oil, avocados, bell peppers, soybeans, flaxseed, Brussels sprouts, legumes, apples, red wine, coffee, tea, vegetable juices, whole grains, and plant sterols and stanols found in enriched orange juice and butter-like spreads. Soy products, with high levels of phytoestrogens, may be better than hormone replacements. The Okinawans, with the highest percentage of centenarians, eat an average of three ounces of soy products per day with the largest source being tofu.

Oily or fatty cold-water fish like salmon, herring, trout, mackerel, anchovies, and sardines may have a special status in the "superfood" department. The two

Table 4. Omega-3 fatty acids in Seafood Sources

Fish	Grams of Omega-3 Fatty Acids per 100-gm (3.5 oz) Serving
Herring	2.1 – 2.2
Salmon	1.8 – 2.3 (lox = 0.5)
Sardines (canned)	1.5 – 1.6
Mackerel	1.5 – 1.9 (king mackerel = 0.4)
Trout	1.1 – 1.2
Halibut	0.5 – 1.2 (Greenland halibut high)
Tuna (fresh)	0.3 – 1.5 (bluefin high; skipjack, yellowfin low)
Shrimp (canned)	0.6
Flounder/Sole	0.5
Crab	0.4 – 0.5
Scallops	0.4
Shrimp (fresh)	0.3
Catfish	0.3 – 0.5
Tuna (canned)	0.2 – 0.4
Cod	0.2 – 0.3
Lobster (northern)	0.1

omega-3 polyunsaturated fatty acids, eicosapentaenoic acid (EPA) and docosahexaenoic acid (DHA), which are found in the oil of these fish, have remarkable health-enhancing properties as demonstrated in numerous studies. EPA and DHA help stabilize cell membranes, are the building blocks for hormones, lower the risk for blood clots, improve arterial elasticity, help maintain normal heartbeat rhythms, lower triglycerides, stabilize arterial plaques, improve endothelial function of the arteries, and reduce inflammation throughout the body. Studies have shown that omega-3 fatty acids lower the risk of heart attacks, stroke, and Alzheimer's disease (Daviglus et al, 1997; Hu et al, 2002, Albert et al, 2002; Morris et al, 2003; Robinson and Stone, 2006).

Oily or fatty cold-water fish like salmon, herring, trout, mackerel, anchovies, and sardines may have a special status in the "superfood" department.

Unfortunately, the American diet is usually deficient in EPA and DHA, raising the risk for these life-shortening diseases. The AHA, American Stroke Association, and Alzheimer's Association all recommend that healthy people eat two fatty or oily fish meals per week to lower the risk of these diseases (Kris-Etherton et al, 2003). Taking fish oil supplements may also help lower risk of these and other disorders, but should not be taken without first consulting with a physician. Major fish sources of the omega-3 fatty acids with amounts per serving are shown in *Table 4* (Finfish and Shellfish Products, USDA National Nutrient Database for Stand Reference, Release 19, 2006).

Getting a sufficient amount of protein, calcium, and vitamin D is also a key factor in achieving centenarian status. Older people may consume lower amounts of protein-rich foods like fish and poultry, causing deficiencies in intake of essential amino acids and vitamin B_{12}. In the Japanese Centenarian Study, a more frequent intake of protein was associated with centenarians who were still able to live independently compared to other elderly people (Ozaki et al, 2006). Okinawan centenarians have high levels of calcium in their diets, and vitamin D from both their diets and sun exposure, resulting in very low levels of osteoporosis and bone fractures compared to other Americans. In the U.S., four out of five osteoporosis diagnoses are in women, and there are more than 1.3 million osteoporotic factures each year, mostly in women. Such fractures can lead to a loss of function and frailty and, in the case of hip fractures, even loss of life.

Eating a fiber-rich breakfast appears to be an important factor in longevity. Ferrucci and colleagues in the Baltimore Longitudinal Study of Aging found that a serving of whole grains, especially in the morning, appears to help older individuals maintain stable blood sugar levels throughout the day and lower their incidence of diabetes—a known accelerator of aging.

Even eating chocolate may have some health and longevity benefits. Now, there's a good research finding! Certain kinds of chocolate may have high levels of flavonols that some studies have found to increase arterial blood flow and reduce inflammation. Although chocolate contains three saturated fats, two of these three fats either don't raise blood cholesterol or help to slightly lower it. But don't stuff a handful of chocolates in your mouth just yet—there are some caveats. The chocolate must be relatively unprocessed dark chocolate (typically 70 percent cacao or greater) and the amount consumed daily for the health benefit is only about the size of a couple of Hershey's kisses. Go over that size and the high sugar/fat intake begins to counteract the benefit.

Centenarians also appear to have higher intakes of coffee than seen in the general American population. A number of studies have found those who drink three to five cups of coffee per day compared to those who drink less have generally better brain and body functioning and lower rates of heart attacks, strokes, diabetes, Alzheimer's disease, and Parkinson's disease (Andersen et al, 2006). This may be due to a combination of the caffeine content and its mild diuretic effect, phenolic antioxidants, and anti-inflammatory effect. One exception may be unfiltered coffee drinks like espresso and "French-press" coffee which may raise LDL cholesterol levels. Tea (whether white, green, oolong, or black) also has powerful levels of polyphenol antioxidants. All these teas are derived from the leaves of the same plant, *camellia sinensis*. The only difference is when the leaves are picked and how much they are processed and oxidized (called fermentation). Green tea has about 10 percent more antioxidants than the most-oxidized tea, black tea. Many Japanese and Okinawan centenarians drink several cups of tea daily.

Step 7: Take Your Vitamins

A large body of research indicates that oxidative stress from free radical damage contributes to aging and the development of age-related diseases that shorten life. Vitamins and antioxidant enzymes have a fundamental role in boosting the immune system and defending the human body from free-radical damage. There are 13 micronutrient substances necessary for good physiological functioning that we call vitamins: the group of eight B vitamins and vitamins A, C, D, E, and K. Centenarians generally have been found to have high blood levels of vitamins, especially A and E (Meccoci et al, 2000). Much of this comes from the vitamin-rich vegetables and fruits that form such a large part of a typical centenarian diet. Vitamins can also be obtained from multivitamin supplements. Many centenarians in western countries have taken a multivitamin on a daily or every-other-day basis for many years.

There is still some argument in the medical and nutritional fields about whether or not to take a daily multivitamin in order to ensure adequate levels of vitamins in the body. Long-term randomized controlled trials are hard to do with vitamins, but the longest studies have suggested that taking a daily multivitamin may help avoid problems from vitamin deficiencies during aging. Many people over age 60 years are vitamin-deficient, with negative health consequences. As we age, it becomes more and more difficult to absorb some essential vitamins such as B_{12} and some minerals from the diet and, the trend found in long-term studies is that multivitamin/multimineral supplementation may be beneficial in achieving an optimal level of health and longevity. The Harvard aging studies, directed by Dr. Walter Willett, have suggested that taking a multivitamin each day makes it more likely one will live longer and healthier (Willett, 2001). Susan Bowerman, MS, RD, of the UCLA Center for Human Nutrition says, "Everyone in the over-60 group should take a multiple vitamin/mineral supplement because, as people get older, their diets may not be as well balanced as they once were, or they take in less food in an effort to control weight in the face of declining metabolic rates." As always, see your doctor before beginning to take any vitamins or other supplements.

Some particular vitamins are candidates for individual supplementation. A panel of the National Institutes of Health estimates that 90 percent of adults between the ages of 51 and 70 years are deficient in vitamin D. Vitamin D is the only vitamin that can be produced in the body—in response to the exposure of skin to sunlight. Unfortunately, the amount of vitamin D made by the body in response to sunlight declines with advancing age. Low vitamin D levels increases the risk for many age-related diseases like cancer, hypertension, diabetes, osteoporosis, and autoimmune diseases. People in the northern or southern latitudes may have especially low levels of vitamin D, and this vitamin must be obtained in the form of a supplement. Vitamin D is especially important for bone health and avoiding fractures. Okinawan centenarians have high levels of vitamin D probably due to their lifetime regular sun exposure and Okinawans in general have one-half the number of hip fractures of Americans. Vitamin D supplementation is recommended for many Americans. Adults should get 400 IUs daily, while people age 71 years and older need even more— 1000 IUs per day.

Calcium is another nutrient that may need to be supplemented, especially for post-menopausal women. Many experts recommend taking 1,200 mg of calcium with vitamin D supplementation to get optimal bone health. Splitting the calcium into two doses of 600 mg each may allow for better absorption. Calcium is also necessary for good muscular function and blood pressure normalization. Fish oil, glucosamine and chondroitin, and coenzyme Q_{10} (for some who are taking statin drugs) are other supplements that may be appropriate for use by some individuals after consultation with their physician.

How about specific "anti-aging" supplements that are advertised in the media? There is, at this time, little convincing evidence that these "anti-aging" remedies, medicines, or hormone treatments have any affect on either slowing the aging process or increasing the chances of becoming a healthy centenarian (Butler et al, 2002). Much of this appears to be quackery practiced in "anti-aging" clinics and falsely advertised in newspapers, magazines, TV, radio, and on the internet. For example, there is no evidence that human growth hormone supplementation enhances healthy life expectancies or the chances of achieving centenarian status (Perls, 2004; Perls, Reisman, and Olshansky, 2005). Since dietary and herbal supplements are unregulated the FDA since the 1994 Dietary Supplements Health and Education Act, some forms of inadequately-researched "anti-aging" supplementation may even be dangerous to health. Dr. Andrew Weil, the well-known integrative medicine practitioner, warns consumers to beware of "anti-aging" supplements and, instead, construct a lifestyle that lowers the risk of major disease threats and achieves optimal physical and mental health. Few, if any, centenarians have been found who have taken these "anti-aging" supplements, which should tell us something about their impact on living a long and healthy life.

Step 8: Exercise Regularly, Be Active, and Stay Busy After Retirement

"Exercise is the only real fountain of youth that exists," says S. Jay Olshansky, PhD, a professor of medicine and researcher on aging at the University of Illinois in Chicago. Although there are thousands of medications and herbal supplements available today for treating various ailments and promoting health, none of them can deliver all the beneficial effects of regular exercise. Across all studies, centenarians tend to have a lifelong history of regular physical activity. They regularly exercise and maintain an active lifestyle for as long as they are able. This is one of the most powerful predictors of successful aging, because lack of exercise is a powerful risk factor for developing heart disease, stroke, many cancers, diabetes, Alzheimer's disease, and many other age-related disorders. Getting regular exercise improves the chances of avoiding all of these diseases and having a long and healthy life.

Centenarians tend to have a lifelong history of regular physical activity.

Unfortunately, only about 25 percent of Americans exercise regularly, and just 10 percent of those over age 65 years get rigorous exercise on a regular basis. Exercise and physical fitness may even be more important in longevity than maintaining a normal body weight (Ming Wei et al, 1999; Church et al, 2005). The Cooper Institute and Aerobics Center Longitudinal Study found increased fitness to be associated with reduced death rates in all weight categories—normal, overweight, and obese. In fact, an overweight individual who exercised regularly outlived a normal-weight individual who did not exercise.

Regular exercise becomes more and more important as the body ages, especially after age 70 years. Sedentary people lose approximately 40 percent of muscle mass and 30 percent of strength between the ages of 20 and 70 years, in part because of a lack of exercise. Between the ages of 20 and 70 years, aerobic capacity declines at a rate of about six percent per decade. However, after age 70 years, body fitness undergoes accelerated decline at a rate of about 20 percent per decade. Without being fit, bodies are too weak to fight off infections, recover from a heart attack or stroke, or survive a fall. It was thought for many years that older people naturally lost muscle mass and became physically frail, and that there was nothing to be done about it. Research now tells us just the opposite. Significant levels of resistance exercise in extremely old age can counteract the natural decline in body functioning and prevent loss of muscle tissue. Those people who do not exercise regularly become decrepit and frail, making them prone to all kinds of aging complications by the time they reach 80 years of age. In particular, life-shortening and disabling falls in old age can be prevented by regular resistance training exercises. Avoiding physical frailty is a key to becoming a centenarian. With a good exercise regimen, a fit 70-year-old can be in better physical shape than the average college student.

Resistance exercise can build and maintain good muscle mass at advanced ages—even past age 100 years. The New England Centenarian Study found that all their healthy centenarians had a full day of activity each and every day (Perls et al, 1999). Many of these 100-year-olds lived on the second or third floors and regularly climbed these stairs for daily exercise. Regular exercise was found to be especially prevalent in those who were still living independently (Ozaki et al, 2006). Centenarians are active and vigorous walkers, bikers, swimmers, gardeners, and golfers. In Okinawa, centenarians regularly do tai chi and karate. The benefits of regular exercise include better cardiovascular health, improved mood, better mental acuity, better balance and fewer falls, greater muscle mass, and better bone density. One man in the New

England Centenarian Study shoots an average golf score of 85, recently won his club's 55-and-older tournament, and can drive his three-wood over 180 yards—at 102 years of age. Being old doesn't mean you have to be physically frail.

Many of the current centenarians grew up in an era when physical labor was a big part of life. They didn't have the plethora of labor-saving devices that permeate our culture now. The active physical lifestyles of their youth and middle age seem to have carried over into old age, as current centenarians continue their habits of doing regular daily physical activities that require exercise and promote general health. However, physical activity has declined precipitously in current young and middle-aged Americans compared to just a few decade ago, which could lower the odds of today's young people becoming centenarians. Lack of exercise contributes to an increased chance of developing cardiovascular disease, diabetes, and many cancers— diseases that shorten American life expectancies. If this trend continues, it could possibly indicate that the number of centenarians predicted in the future may not be as high as we think.

Three-fourths of Americans do not exercise regularly. The greatest benefit for health and the slowing of aging for the average American is going from being sedentary to just walking briskly for 30 minutes three to four times a week on a regular basis.. Daily exercise is even better. Nearly all studies agree that getting a good "moderate" intensity cardiovascular workout is key. But, what exactly is a "moderate" exercise level? San Diego State University researcher Simon Marshall, in a May, 2009 *American Journal of Preventive Medicine* study, outlined some practical ways to determine this. By studying 97 healthy men and women, three criteria emerged that are useful to the average person. First, when walking, about 100 steps per minute is a moderate exercise level and a good general target. Men in the study got to a moderate intensity level with 92 to 102 steps per minute, while women did it in 91 to 115 steps. (Steps per minute can be measured by counting with a watch or using a cheap pedometer that measures steps.) Second, you can count your heartbeats per minute. Moderate exercise is when the heart rate is between 50 percent and 85 percent of the maximum heart rate (calculated by subtracting your age from 220). Third, the "talk test," can be used. You are exercising at a moderate intensity level when you are breathing faster than normal but can still say a sentence or two or sing a bit of a favorite song. You should be out of breath after doing either, and if you are not, you are walking at low intensity. If you have trouble finishing a sentence, you are exercising at high intensity.

Strength-building resistance exercises like climbing stairs or lifting light weights are especially beneficial since they slow age-related loss of muscle mass and bone. Water exercises can be very helpful if an individual has arthritis and joint pain. Having a busy, active lifestyle may be more important than sporadic visits to the gym. Building in regular things into your daily routine like taking the stairs instead of the elevator, parking the car farther from a destination, taking a walking break instead of a coffee break, planning active vacations, and just walking every day is what seems to work for centenarians. Huffing and puffing at the gym is fine, but is not necessary. Only a small percentage of centenarians ever had a gym membership.

Weight-resistant exercise also helps bones stay dense and strong. Along with diets high in calcium and high vitamin D synthesis from sun exposure, this helps Okinawan centenarians avoid bone fractures, especially disastrous hip fractures that are often associated with shortened life spans in the elderly. Okinawans exercise more than Americans. Okinawans, with longer life spans and higher percentages of centenarians, have about 50 percent fewer hip fractures than Americans (Ross et al, 1991). Suzuki and colleagues, in the 1995 *Journal of Bone Research*, demonstrated that Okinawan centenarians preserve their bone densities for longer periods of time than other Japanese. Frail musculature from lack of exercise can be a major cause of falls and bone fractures that can markedly reduce the level of self-care. In the Japanese Centenarian Study, not having severe falls after age 95 years strongly predicted who would still live independently after age 100 years (Ozaki et al, 2006). Exercising and staying strong is a major characteristic of successful aging.

Avoiding inactive retirement and having a busy lifestyle also appear to be factors in reaching the oldest ages. "Evidence shows that in societies where people stop working abruptly, the incidence of obesity and chronic disease skyrockets after retirement," says Luigi Ferrucci, M.D., Ph.D., director of the Baltimore Longitudinal Study of Aging. The New England Centenarian Study found that centenarians typically live surprisingly productive lives and wake up each day with eager anticipation to get things done (Perls et al, 1999). Retirement doesn't have to be sedentary. For example, in the Chianti region of Italy, which has a high percentage of centenarians, retirement is different. Here, Dr. Ferrucci says, "After people retire from their jobs, they spend most of the day working on their little farm, cultivating grapes or vegetables—they are never really inactive." The idea of retirement seems never to have occurred to Okinawan centenarians. To this day, there is not a word for retirement in the Okinawan language. It appears that staying busy and active every day is a very important predictor of becoming a centenarian.

Step 9: Don't Smoke or Stop Smoking If You Do

Very few centenarians (less than two percent in many studies) have smoked tobacco (Poon et al, 1992;

Zyczkowska et al, 2006). Nearly all of them have not smoked at all in their lives and, among those few centenarians who did smoke, they did not smoke for a long period of time before quitting (Perls et al, 1999). These findings are based on large groups of centenarians. There are always some rare exceptions to the rule. For example, the longest-lived documented person in history, Jeanne Calment, smoked from adolescence until she was 117 years of age. That makes her an extreme rarity for a centenarian. It is important to remember that smoking is associated with high levels of heart disease, cancer, stroke, lung disease, and other life-threatening illnesses, as well as Alzheimer's disease. Most regular smokers will not live long, healthy lives.

Smoking is the most important behavioral health hazard and the single most preventable cause of death and disease for Americans. Cigarette smoke contains toxins that directly damage DNA and subsequently cause many cancers. Nitrosamines and other substances in cigarette smoke are potent oxidants and carcinogens that lead to accelerated aging and diseases associated with aging. Over 400,000 people die annually in the U.S. from smoking-related diseases. According to the American Cancer Society, smoking has been linked to at least 10 different types of cancer and accounts for 30 percent of all cancer deaths. What most people don't know is that most smokers die of heart disease. Toxins from tobacco smoke in the bloodstream damage the endothelium or arteries and help start the accumulation of atherosclerotic plaque in the arteries. Smoking is a contributing factor in 40 percent of all deaths from heart disease and stroke, the first and third leading causes of death. Smoking is also the major cause of the fourth leading cause of death, COPD.

> **Smoking is the most important behavioral health hazard and the single most preventable cause of death and disease for Americans.**

Cigarette smoking is the most deadly type of smoking. Basically, every cigarette smoked takes an average of seven minutes off your life. The average individual who begins smoking in adolescence and continues smoking throughout their lives loses about 7 to 13 years of life expectancy, depending on numbers of cigarettes smoked per day. Obviously, this markedly reduces the chance that a smoker will make it to 100 years of age. Reports from the U.S. Surgeon General state that second-hand smoke from other smokers or air pollution may be 20 to 30 percent as dangerous to health as cigarette smoking itself.

If you smoke, quitting may be the single most important thing you can do to increase the odds of a long and healthy life. Quitting smoking reduces heart disease risk within a few years and, within 10 to 15 years, former smokers' lung cancer risk is close to those who have never smoked. Smoking is a powerful addiction due to the effects of nicotine. Unfortunately, U.S. smoking rates have stabilized in the last few years at about 22 percent after falling for several decades. Men are more likely to smoke. However, women are more likely to be addicted to nicotine, and the number of adolescent female smokers appears to be increasing in recent years. Most smokers quit without any formal program, although it often takes many attempts to do so. Many programs are available for those who cannot stop smoking on their own. Many have both psychological therapies and medical components such as nicotine replacement and medications like *varenicline tartrate* (Chantix®) and *buproprion* (Wellbutrin®). The bottom line is, if you want to be a healthy centenarian, don't smoke or, if you do, quit as soon as you can.

Step 10: Drink Less Alcohol

Alcohol and aging represent an interesting conundrum. The average American drinks about 2.3 gallons of pure alcohol per year. Since about 70 percent of American men and 60 percent of women drink, the average drinker probably imbibes nearly three gallons per year. So, is this too much? It's a difficult question to answer simply. Dozens of studies have shown that "moderate" alcohol consumption seems to protect against heart disease and stroke—the leading killer of Americans. Worldwide studies have found that moderate drinking increases HDL cholesterol, reduces blood clots, makes blood vessel walls less vulnerable to atherosclerosis, raises omega-3 fatty acids in the blood, increases bone density, and reduces the risk for Alzheimer's disease and vascular dementia. AHA guidelines currently state that moderate alcohol consumption, for the average American reduces the risk of heart disease and ischemic strokes—the most common kind. The AHA guidelines are: for women, one drink per day; for men, one to two drinks per day. A drink is defined as a 12-ounce beer, 4 ounces of wine, and 1.5 ounces of 80-proof liquor (about a shot glass filled to the top). Women must drink less because of their smaller bodies and blood volume and lower amounts of enzymes that break down alcohol. It should be understood that exceeding these levels—even by *one* drink per day— *increases* the risk for heart disease, stroke, liver disease, and some cancers. So, there is a very narrow window for any benefit. It is important to realize that the alcohol benefit for increased life expectancy exists for the average American, who is somewhat overweight, has slightly elevated LDL cholesterol and slightly low HDL cholesterol, has slightly elevated trigylcerides, and has a blood pressure of about 130/80, which is pre-hypertensive.

So, will that daily glass of red wine help get you to 100 years old? Overall, it seems not to be an important factor for centenarians. Actually, most centenarians have not drunk much alcohol at all. The New England Centenarian Study found that alcohol consumption

> **Most centenarians have not drunk much alcohol at all.**

was extremely uncommon among centenarians (Perls et al, 1999). Only a very few drank regularly. The Japanese Centenarian Study found that having no history of drinking alcohol was a strong predictor of independent-living after age 100 (Ozaki et al, 2006). In the National Institute of Mental Health aging studies, 80 percent of those reaching 100 years of age had consumed less than one alcoholic drink per month. The "Blue Zone" Seventh Day Adventist centenarians around Loma Linda, California have abstained from alcohol completely. True, men in the "Blue Zone" of Sardinia who have remarkably long life spans and high percentage of centenarians drink a couple of glasses of wine a day. However, the vast majority of centenarians in studies around the world consumed alcohol only occasionally, if at all.

On the whole, if you want to be a centenarian and have a healthy lifestyle, it may be helpful to drink less or not at all. One drink a day for a woman and one to two drinks for a man may be healthy and extend life slightly for "average" Americans (who won't reach

100 years) because of their somewhat elevated levels of LDL cholesterol, blood pressure, blood sugar, and triglyceride levels. However, this is not the common practice of centenarians. In any case, there are always exceptions. The longest-lived individual in recent times, Jeanne Calment, was reported to have consumed a glass of port with lunch and a glass of wine with dinner starting in her early teens and continuing over her life until just a few days before she died. One thing is pretty evident: if you drink to excess beyond one drink a day for a woman and two for a man, you are severely limiting your chances of reaching 100 years of age. So, alcohol appears to be a double-edged sword in the aging process—good if you are at some risk for life-shortening disease but not especially helpful if you have an otherwise healthy lifestyle.

Step 11: Get Regular and Restful Sleep

Sleep is crucial for good health. Regular and restful sleep helps keep immune systems strong, keep blood pressure and blood sugar at low levels, resist weight gain and obesity, assist in emotional stability and forming new memories, and reduce pain perception.

Centenarians typically have regular sleep patterns and get plenty of restful, restorative sleep.

Many older people in their 70s and 80s get only about six hours of sleep per night. Centenarians typically have regular sleep patterns and get plenty of restful, restorative sleep—usually seven to eight hours. One of the major characteristics of 100-year-olds in the Costa Rican "Blue Zone" was sleeping about eight hours per day on a regular basis (Buettner, 2008). While sleep times can vary from person to person, getting the regular rest is the key. Centenarians have established sleep routines, tending to go to bed and wake up at the same time each day. In general, they go to sleep when the sun goes down and wake up when it comes up. In the Japanese Centenarian Study, spontaneously waking up at regular times in the morning was a major characteristic of those who were living independently (Ozaki et al, 2006).

Taking a nap during the day may be a healthy sleeping pattern for older people. While sleeping continuously throughout the night is often touted as the most recommended way to sleep, midday napping appears to be a common characteristic of the healthiest older people. In the MEDIS study of long-lived people in the Mediterranean islands (Tourlouki et al, 2009), all of the people in the study older than 90 years were found to engage in naps around noontime.

Unfortunately, as many as 40 percent of the elderly have some type of sleep disorder that can result in physical and cognitive problems. "Short-sleepers" getting less than six hours of sleep a night have been found to have poor insulin control of blood sugar, more diabetes and obesity, stronger appetites, more heart attacks, and shorter life spans. These risks are even more pronounced for those getting five or less hours of sleep per night. Obesity and sleep deprivation are strongly connected. Studies show that, compared to those getting about eight hours of sleep per night, those who sleep only five hours have a 50 percent higher chance of becoming obese. Those who sleep only four hours have a 73 percent higher chance of obesity. It also appears that getting too much sleep—*hypersomnia*—of nine or more hours nightly may be even worse for health and longevity than sleep deprivation.

Increasing age increases the chance of developing several sleep disorders. Sleep disorders are associated with many health problems and are major risk factors for heart disease, stroke, depression, and even Alzheimer's disease. Common age-related sleep disorders include insomnia, obstructive sleep disorder, restless legs, periodic limb movement disorder, and REM behavior disorder. Insomnia is the biggest culprit, because it is the most common sleep disorder. Other less-common sleep disorders may be even more dangerous. Obstructive sleep apnea, for example, dramatically raises the risk of heart attack and stroke. According to a study in the November, 2008 *American Journal of Respiratory and Critical Care*, even mild obstructive sleep apnea raises cardiovascular disease risk because of increased arterial stiffness. It seems clear that getting a good night's sleep is crucial to health and longevity.

If there are problems sleeping, there are techniques you can try at home to help, called "sleep hygiene." Techniques of improving sleep with easily-implemented sleep hygiene strategies can be found on the internet, and many people can help themselves to a better night's sleep by using them. Centenarians practice many of these techniques. If sleep hygiene techniques do not work and sleep problems continue, the best recommendation is to see a sleep disorders specialist or go to a sleep disorders clinic for thorough evaluation, diagnosis, and treatment. Bottom line: to live long, sleep well.

Step 12: Maintain Healthy Gums

Avoiding gum disease in the form of mild gingivitis to more severe periodontitis lowers the risk of age-related diseases and is associated with longer life expectancy. Gum disease results from bacterial infections. Studies have found that those people with the highest amounts of bacteria in their mouths are the most likely to have thickening of the arteries in the form of atherosclerotic plaque—a major risk factor for heart attack and stroke. Low-grade, chronic inflammation from such gum infections appears to be the culprit.

There is an old saying: "We dig our graves with our teeth." Having healthy gums is associated with the retention of teeth over the years. A number of participants in the New England Centenarian Study

"We dig our graves with our teeth."

were found to still have all their teeth, which is not all that unusual for this group. In the Japanese Centenarian Study, one of the major characteristics of independent-living 100-year-olds is that they were still able to effectively masticate their food. Keeping gums is healthy and free of inflammation one of the key contributors to long and healthy life spans. Brushing and flossing teeth regularly reduces the amount of gum-disease-causing bacteria in the mouth, which can enter the bloodstream and trigger inflammation in the arteries. Thomas Perls, of the New England Centenarian Study, states that, "I really do think people should floss twice a day to get the biggest life expectancy benefits."

Step 13: Challenge Your Mind

It is a common belief that the oldest old just sit around, stare into space, and aren't interested in anything. As shown by the New England Centenarian Study and many others, nothing could be further from the truth (Perls et al, 1999). Continued involvement in stimulating, challenging, and interesting mental activities characterizes these "oldest old" centenarians. They read, paint, play musical instruments, learn new languages, and continue to learn and exercise their brains. This appears to build and expand neuronal networks in the brain. As a group, they seem to have retained very good thinking skills. A number of studies have shown that just keeping your mind busy and learning new things markedly reduces the chances of being diagnosed with Alzheimer's disease or, at least, delays this diagnosis through a "cognitive reserve." Higher brain activity and new learning cause growth and connections among the brain's cells that appear more resistant to brain aging. Especially among older men, decreased mental activities results in earlier death. It may be that our love affair with a "laid-back" retirement may be a mixed blessing. Having an active schedule, daily goals, and a purpose to one's existence may be a key to successful aging. Many centenarians continue to stay mentally active on a daily basis by working or volunteering.

Whether formal education is a major predictor of reaching 100 years old is more debatable. In the Georgia Centenarian Study, centenarians who lived independently had higher levels of education than the average American. In this group, higher educational levels seemed to predict better coping skills, overall higher levels of challenging mental activity, and more new learning in the oldest old that were associated with their long-term survival and independence. On the other hand, the average educational level in the New England Centenarian Study was not correlated with achieving extreme old age. In this study, formal education did not seem to have a great effect in helping these people to live to be 100 years old with good cognitive and physical health.

> **Keeping mentally busy and continuing to learn things is important to long-term survival.**

One thing seems to be clear: keeping mentally busy and continuing to learn things is important to long-term survival. No one is quite sure how or why it works, but keeping the mind busy, continuing to learn throughout one's lifetime, and retaining good cognitive abilities all predict the achievement of centenarian status. As summarized by Perls et al. (1999), "It is cognitive capacity, more than any physical disability, that most often determines whether people can attain extreme old age while remaining active…No one achieves extreme old age without retaining a great deal of cognitive ability for the most of his or her life."

Step 14: Stay Positive in Attitude and Avoid Anxiety & Depression

Several studies have found that centenarians have lower levels of tension, anxiety, and depression than other less-older persons. The absence of depression is particularly evident. In a major National Institutes of Mental Health study of aging, less than two percent of 90- and 100-year-olds had ever had any lengthy depression or anxiety disorders. In the Georgia Centenarian study, none of the 100-year-olds who lived independently were found to have any significant clinical depression. In the New England Centenarian Study, only four of 74 centenarians showed signs of clinical depression on the Geriatric Depression Scale (a standardized questionnaire). Importantly, however, none of these four showed any classic symptoms of depression when they were evaluated. Studies show that, if depression episodes had happened sometime during the lives of centenarians, these episodes were short-lived and usually a temporary sadness or bereavement. Centenarians do not avoid grieving after a loss, but go through it, conclude it, and go on with the business of living.

A good way *not* to become a centenarian is to have chronic depression. Chronic depression is a killer—on average, people with chronic depression die years earlier than non-depressed people. Numerous studies have demonstrated that chronic depression and many anxiety disorders are major risk factors for heart disease, stroke, diabetes, and some types of cancer. If depression and anxiety disorders occur, it is important to treat them quickly and effectively to reduce the powerful negative effects on health. Some centenarians had episodes of depression or anxiety, but tended to recover quickly and move on. Fortunately, the National Institute of Mental Health states that the treatment success for major depressive disorder is 80 percent if there are persistent interventions with antidepressant medications, psychotherapy, repetitive transcranial magnetic stimulation, vagal stimulation, deep brain stimulation, and electroconvulsive therapy.

Anxiety disorders can be treated successfully in 70 to 90 percent of cases, depending upon the particular disorder, by medication and psychotherapy. It appears that either avoiding or quickly and effectively treating any depression and anxiety disorder that occurs is an important part of making it to 100 years old.

All studies have found that centenarians are typically positive, happy, and extremely satisfied with their lives. For example, researches found Costa Rican centenarians to be extremely positive about their lives. Many studies have found a connection between optimism and long lives. The 100,000 women aged 50 years and older in the Women's Health Initiative (WHI) have been followed with various studies since 1994. In this group, researchers found those with optimistic attitudes lived longer and healthier lives than more pessimistic women. During eight years of follow-up, WHI optimists were 30 percent less likely to die of heart disease and 14 percent less likely to die of any cause compared

> **Centenarians are typically positive, happy, and extremely satisfied with their lives.**

to pessimists. Another 2004 study that looked at longevity among more than 900 older adults found those who were optimistic had a 29 percent lower risk of early death than the pessimists. A Milwaukee study of the Catholic sisters of Notre Dame found that the number of times the nuns used positive and negative words dramatically affected their life expectancy. These nuns had remarkably similar routines and lifestyles. However, two-thirds of the nuns using negative words often died before their 85th birthday. Among the positive nuns, 90 percent of them were still alive at age 85 years, and outlived their negative sisters by about nine years. Centenarians have positive and optimistic attitudes about themselves and their lives, and have a high level of self-confidence.

Pessimism and negative thinking are seldom seen in centenarians. As summarized by Dr. Perls, "Personality is one of the most important factors in survival" (Perls et al, 1999). In the New England Centenarian Study, 100-year-olds had low levels of unhealthy "neuroticism," i.e., negative emotional feelings like anger, fear, guilt, and sadness that are associated with depression and anxiety disorders. Anxious and fearful thoughts can negatively impact health status. Pessimistic attitudes are associated with high disease rates and shorter life spans. In a Mayo Clinic study following 7,000 people over four decades, the most pessimistic, anxious, and depressed people had a 30 percent greater chance of dying than those who were most optimistic, least anxious, and least depressed. The low "neuroticism" of centenarians means that they are calm and collected, with fewer extreme negative emotional reactions, even during crises. They simply have chosen to think in a positive manner rather than a negative one. One of the participants in the New England study said her philosophy of life was, "Pick out the fine things in life, and if you can't find them there, pick them out of your own head." (Perls et al, 1999). So, work on staying positive and upbeat about life—it's a way to live longer and better.

Emotional stability is also important. Centenarians seem to have had stable personalities throughout their lives, with low levels of negative thoughts, emotions, and moods. As noted by Perls et al (1999), "Perhaps maintaining emotional stability in old age is much more crucial for long-term physical and cognitive health than is currently given credit for." As they get older, centenarians' personalities become even more consistent and less variable in conduct and moods. They are less likely to have mood swings or become anxious or depressed as they age. In general, centenarians are emotionally stable, flexible, and adaptive. Although subjected to multiple separations and bereavements at the highest age levels, they endure, cope well, and even flourish as a result. Centenarians become the ultimate physical survivors, in large part because of their remarkable emotional stability.

Step 15: Shed Those Stressors, Have Daily Structure, and Be Resilient

Personality can be defined as one's patterns of behavior and various habitual methods of adjusting to life's demands. Positive personality traits are a strong indicator of living to very old age. In fact, Dr. Perls of the New England Centenarian Study believes that personality is the most important factor in the longevity of centenarians. How one handles stress is an important part of personality and has a profound effect on life expectancy. In particular, how someone thinks about and copes with negative environmental stressors like jobs, the death of loved ones, marital difficulties, and ongoing life challenges

> **How one handles stress is an important part of personality and has a profound effect on life expectancy.**

is an extremely important predictor of who will make it to 100 years old.

Stress usually happens when we have difficulty coping with negative factors in the environment. In other words, we stress ourselves by what we think about negative stressors. We've known this for 2,000 years, going back to the Greek stoic philosopher Epictitus, who said, "We are not disturbed by things, but by our *perception* of things." Centenarians just don't seem to stress themselves as much or as often as most people do. The Swedish Centenarian Study found those who were less prone to anxiety and worrying were much more likely to make it to 100 years old (Samuelsson et al, 1997). Across all studies that measured stress, centenarians seem to have life-long stable personalities that seem to shed stress (called "teflon personalities" by some). They have low levels of stress and an easy-going approach to life, which is often the result of conscious decisions. As one individual in the New England Centenarian Study stated, "I decided not to worry about anything....I saw that worrying didn't do any good" (Perls et al, 1999). Avoiding the worrying of chronic stress is a key to successful aging. Chronic stress is a killer of the body and brain. Researcher Jay Olshansky calls chronic emotional stress an "aging accelerator" that shortens life and markedly reduces the odds of becoming a centenarian.

It was previously thought that centenarians had low levels of stress because they somehow avoided the negative stressors in life, like they avoided the common diseases of aging. However, when centenarians are asked if they had a lot of stress in their lives, they usually answered "yes." Studies show that centenarians have been exposed to as many environmental stressors as the rest of us, surviving losses of many loved ones and living through harsh times like the Great Depression (Perls et al, 1999). Some have even been survivors of extreme stress situations like Nazi concentration camps during World War II. Being open and extroverted, centenarians seem to effectively handle environmental stressors and deal with life's ongoing problems with cognitive coping skills as they occur—and then move on with their lives (Martin et al, 1992; Masul et al, 2006). Many make comments like, "I dealt with it, got over it, and didn't let it bother me a lot after that." They have a remarkable capacity for coping with the stress of separation and bereavement—which has usually happened several times—and continue to maintain their emotional focus and concentrate on survival (Perls et al, 1999). Clearly, holding on to negative memories and remaining upset by them is not seen much in these oldest old.

Centenarians are resilient. As noted by Dr. Thomas Perls, "We have a new study coming out that shows that centenarians tend not to internalize things or dwell on their troubles. They are great at rolling with the punches." Centenarians tend to be decisive, know what they want, and stay on course. However, when life circumstances force them to adapt, they become flexible thinkers and are able to embrace change. They adapt, cope, and move on. Extreme longevity is not about avoiding life's problems, but rather responding to them efficiently and effectively.

Successfully coping with negative stressors is a powerful predictor of becoming a centenarian. Overall, older men appear to have more stress from jobs and other environmental stressors than women, and this may contribute to the higher numbers of female centenarians in most studies. In cultures where stress appears to be greater in females, they don't live as long as males. For example, one of Dan Buettner's "Blue Zones" with very high percentages of 100-year-olds is in Sardinia. Here, male centenarians outnumber female centenarians—an unusual finding. Buettner observed that women appear to take on most of the stressors in the Sardinian culture, while men had a comparatively more stress-free lifestyle. This seemed to be a major factor in increasing the numbers of male centenarians compared to women.

Centenarians also tend to have a lifestyle characterized by non-stressful behavioral routines, according to Jay Olshansky, Ph.D., a specialist on aging from the University of Chicago. They typically have a very structured day, doing the same activities according to a standard schedule. On a daily basis, they tend to eat the same kind of food, go to sleep and wake up spontaneously at the same times, and do the same kinds of activities over their whole lives. Such routines seem to help with stress reduction. Disruption of these routines in older persons, especially sleep, can have serious consequences. This steady equilibrium of routine lifestyle activities seems to keep centenarians feeling happy, healthy, and grounded.

One stress-shedding personality trait common in centenarians is a good sense of humor. They lighten their emotional load by laughing about it. Even cognitive-impaired centenarians in the New England Study had retained their sense of humor. Humor often helps people deal with physical and psychological pain and allows them to get on with their lives. The physiological afterglow of a good laugh is a relaxed, non-stressful state. Laughing and smiling have been found to have similar physiological benefits as physical exercise such as lower blood pressure and more disease-fighting antibodies in the bloodstream.

One reason that being able to handle stressful aspects of life is a key to longer life is that stress is a major risk factor for heart disease, stroke, cancer, and immune system problems. The importance of effectively dealing with stress cannot be overemphasized. In a large study in Germany, job-related stress was shown to be six times the risk factor for heart disease and cancer than smoking and high cholesterol! This was especially true for those in their 50s and 60s. The pervasive anger and hostility often associated with chronic stress, sometimes called a "Type D Personality," has been found to be a particular indicator of cardiovascular disease and a shortened life expectancy (Denollet et al, 1996, 2000). Chronic stress is also a major cause of anxiety and depression, which have been shown to cause chemical changes and cell damage in the brain that disrupt thought processes and impair the ability of people to manage their lives.

Managing stress is a learned skill, and practicing it effectively is key to a longer, healthier life. Stress management often involves learning to meditate and relax, along with developing new mental strategies for effectively managing life's problems. Yoga, exercise, meditation, tai chi, knitting, or just deep breathing can all be effective stress reducers, depending on the person. Stress-related damage to the body and brain has been linked to chronically high levels of stress hormones like cortisol. Researchers such as Herbert Benson, director of the Mind/Body Medical Institute at Massachusetts General Hospital, have demonstrated that the circulating levels of these stress hormones drop with meditation and relaxation exercises. It's never too late to learn new stress management skills or improve old ones—and it could get you closer to being a healthy, happy 100-year-old.

Step 16: Stay Socially Connected with Serenity and a Purpose to Life

Centenarians generally have open, extroverted personalities (Masul et al, 2006), typically being friendly with others and maintaining close ties with friends and family. Meaningful social relationships are an important survival tool. In the New England Study, despite outliving numerous family members and friends, nearly all centenarians have many meaningful relationships and almost none were "loners." The oldest old who have more social ties have been shown to have lower levels of functional and cognitive decline in a number of studies (Unger et al, 1999; Bassuk, Glass and Berkman, 1999; Aartsen et al, 2005).

Positive social relationships and support systems are associated with lower rates of depression and a longer life. Centenarians tend to be outgoing, socially involved, and get a lot of satisfaction from their relationships with others. Some of the biggest benefits of exercise in centenarians may be a result of the strong social interactions that come from walking with a buddy or doing a group exercise class. Independent, community-dwelling centenarians in the Georgia Centenarian Study were found to have good family social support systems. Centenarians seem to have personalities

> **Nearly all centenarians have many meaningful relationships and almost none were "loners."**

that attract people. Having daily supportive connections with friends and family members seems to give a safe and secure feeling of someone "having your back" (Capurso et al, 1997). It's like a psychological safety net. In Okinawa, centenarians often have a *moai*, a daily ritualized meeting of several close family and/or supportive friends that functions as a vehicle for companionship and communication. Centenarians are almost never lonely, which may help them have a long and healthy life.

Unfortunately, most Americans seem to be increasingly alienated from their neighbors and tend to have only two or three close friends they can count on (Putnam, 2001). This is a clear health risk. Social isolation and loneliness have been linked in numerous studies to cognitive decline, high blood pressure, and the risk of dying from cardiovascular disease. Studies have shown clinically lonely people have systolic blood pressures nearly 30 points higher than people who are not lonely. Loneliness is deadly for both men and women. A nine-year Alameda County, California study of almost 7,000 adults ranging in age from 38 to 94 years found that men with the fewest social and community ties were 2.3 times likely to die as those with the most ties (Berkman and Syme, 1979). The most isolated women were 2.8 times more likely to die than socially-engaged women.

Marital status may be an important contributor to the ability of male centenarians to maintain good cognitive and physical functioning. In the New England

Centenarian Study, 24 percent of men were married (Terry et al, 2008). However, only two percent of female centenarians were married, possibly due to the overall shorter life spans of men they were previously married to. Despite this, 31 percent of males centenarians lived alone compared to 14 percent of females. Compared to men, a surprisingly large percentage of female centenarians had never married. However, even without close family members or children, these lifelong single women were nearly always surrounded by a supportive group of people of all ages.

Centenarians are also characterized by having excellent psychospiritual tranquility and serenity, whether grounded in a religion or just a as a result of a general philosophy of life. A very high level of psychospiritual serenity was found among people in the Okinawa Centenarian Study. As one centenarian in Costa Rica's "Blue Zone" stated, "I have had a tranquil life." (Buettner, 2008, p. 189). Religious beliefs seem to play a particularly strong role in achieving longevity. Studies show that most of the oldest old cite religion in some way as a way of coping with aging, illness, pain, and disability of all kinds. All four centenarian groups in the "Blue Zones" were characterized as having strong religious beliefs: Nicoyan Costa Ricans had a strong

Centenarians are also characterized by having excellent psychospiritual tranquility and serenity.

belief that God would provide, Seventh-Day Adventists had an encompassing Christian faith tradition, Sardinians were devout Catholics, and Okinawans believed that their deceased ancestors watched over them. Religion and frequent prayer have been found in studies to provide important health-giving benefits to older people that often cannot be replicated by drugs or diet. Several studies have found that regular churchgoers live longer, handle stress better, and have lower levels of depression. The Seventh-Day Adventists live nearly 10 years longer than the average American with a philosophy that the body is on loan from God and should be cherished without abuse from smoking, drugs, alcohol, and unhealthy foods. Religious faith among the Adventists seems to provide and maintain a lifestyle with good health habits and great social support among like-minded spiritual people. Being part of God's plan was a key part of centenarians' self-concept in the New England study, allowing them to cope with the inevitability and proximity of death (Perls et al, 1999).

An almost universal finding among centenarians is that they feel that they have a purpose to their lives. They feel that their lives are important and that they have things to do—which they accomplish on a daily basis. This may be a strong contributor to their good self-image and sense of well-being. In Okinawa, they call it *ikigai*—the reason for waking up in the morning. Costa Rican centenarians typically have what they call a *plan de vida*, a strong sense of purpose and a desire to contribute to the greater good that results in their feeling of being needed by others. Centenarians typically get up every day with a purpose, feel that their lives are meaningful, and believe that the direction that their lives take is under their control but guided by an external higher power.

❀ ❀ ❀ ❀ ❀

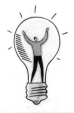

By following the above 16 steps, it is possible to increase the odds that you will live a healthy, happy, and very long life—and even reach 100 years of age. Changing your lifestyle to follow these steps has a dramatic effect on life expectancy. You don't even have to practice them all to get benefits. The supporting data are very clear. To just give four final examples, if you practice just a few of these 16 steps on a consistent basis, your life expectancy is remarkably lengthened.

EXAMPLE 1: You now know that cardiovascular disease—heart attack and stroke—is the biggest threat to having a long and healthy life. A study in the July 2006 journal *Circulation* demonstrated that if you practice only five of the above 16 steps, your risk for cardiovascular disease is vastly reduced. These moderately easily-achieved lifestyle changes are much more important to heart health than taking the statin drugs. If you maintain a healthy weight *(Step 4)*, eat a healthy diet *(Step 6)*, exercise regularly *(Step 8)*, drink alcohol in moderation, if you drink at all *(Step 10)*, and don't smoke *(Step 9)*, the risk of developing heart disease is reduced 87 percent in men and 83 percent in women. That's a huge benefit to life expectancy.

EXAMPLE 2: Could practicing just four of the 16 steps add 14 healthy years to your life expectancy? Look at the 11-year EPIC-Norfolk study that followed 20,244 men and women aged 45 to 79 years and was published in the 2008 *Public Library of Science Medicine* journal by Khaw. This study showed that not smoking *(Step 9)*, drinking moderately *(Step 10)*, keeping physically active *(Step 8)*, and eating five servings of fruits and vegetables daily *(Step 6)* added 14 years to life expectancy compared to people who did not follow any of these steps. As a matter of fact, those people who didn't practice any of these four steps were four times likely to die during the 11-year period than people who did.

EXAMPLE 3: Want a greater than 50 percent chance to live into your 90s? Dr. Laurel Yates and colleagues at Harvard University followed 2,357 men in the 70s for 25 years. In a study published in the *Archives of Internal Medicine* in 2008, if one of these older people regularly practiced just five of the 16 steps—not smoking *(Step 9)*, keeping a normal weight *(Step 4)*, exercising regularly *(Step 8)*, having low blood sugar *(Step 1)*, and having low blood pressure *(Step 2)*—they had a *53 percent chance* of living into their 90s. On the other hand, if they smoked, were obese, were inactive, had diabetes, and had hypertension, there was only a four percent chance of ever getting to 90 years old. As summarized by Dr. Yates, "It's not luck, it's not just genetics…it's lifestyle that seems to make a big difference."

EXAMPLE 4: As shown above in the Harvard study of people in their 70s and 90s, it is never too late to start following the 16 steps if you want a longer, healthier life. And the beneficial effects can be almost immediate, even in older people. In a study at the Medical University of South Carolina published by King in the 2007 *American Journal of Medicine*, people aged 45 to 64 years were followed for four years. Those who practiced four of the 16 steps—eating five

> **If you practice just a few of these 16 steps on a consistent basis, your life expectancy is remarkably lengthened.**

servings of fruits and vegetables daily *(Step 6)*, regularly exercising *(Step 8)*, maintaining a normal body weight *(Step 4)*, and not smoking *(Step 9)*—over the four years reduced their risk for developing cardiovascular disease by 35 percent and their risk for dying by 40 percent.

This course outlines the common 16 lifestyle characteristics of centenarians around the world who often have remarkably intact physical health, mental abilities, and emotional status. They are an amazing group of people. While nothing will guarantee you a long and healthy life, by following these steps, you can boost the odds that you will join this select group and reach 100 years old yourself.

∾ *GOOD LUCK!*

❀ ❀ ❀ ❀ ❀

REFERENCES

1. Aartsen MJ, et al. Does widowhood affect memory performance of older persons? *Psychol Med.* 2005;35(2): 217-226.

2. Aarssen K, de Haan L. On the maximal life span of humans. *Mathematical Population Studies.* 1994;4(4):259-281.

3. Adams ER, et al. Centenarian offspring: Start healthier and stay healthier. *J Am Geriatr Soc.* 2008;56(11): 2089-2092.

4. Albert C, et al. Blood levels of long-chain omega-3 fatty acids and risk of sudden death. *New Engl J Med.* 2002;346: 1113-1118.

5. Albertuzzi P, et al. The effect of dietary soy supplementation on hot flashes. *Obstet Gynecol.* 1998;91:6-11.

6. Allard M, Lebre V, Robine J-M. *Les 120 Ans de Jeanne Calment. Doyenne de L'humanite.* Paris, France: Le Cherche Midi Editeur, 1994.

7. Allard M, Lebre V, Robine J-M, Calment J. *Jeanne Calment: From Van Gogh's Time to Ours: 122 Extraordinary Years.* New York, NY: WH Freeman, 1998.

8. Andersen L, et al. Consumption of coffee is associated with reduced risk of death attributed to inflammatory and cardiovascular disease in the Iowa Women's Health Study. *Am J Clin Nutrition.* 2006;83:1039-1046.

9. Bassuk SS, Glass TA, Berkman LF. Social disengagement and incident cognitive decline in community-dwelling elderly persons. *Ann Intern Med.* 1999;131(3):165-173.

10. Beare S. *50 Secrets of the World's Longest Living People.* Philadelphia, PA: Da Capo Press, Perseus Books Group, 2006.

11. Beers MH (Ed.). *The Merck Manual of Health and Aging.* Whitehouse Station, NJ: Merck Research Laboratories, 2004.

12. Berkman LF, Syme SL. Social networks, host resistance, and mortality: A nine-year follow-up study of Alameda County residents. *Am J Epidemiol.* 1979;109:186-204.

13. Bernstein AM, et al. First autopsy of an Okinawan centenarian: Absence of many age-related diseases. *J Gerontol A Biol Sci Med Sci.* 2004;59(11):1195-1199.

14. Blackwelder WC, Yano K, Rhoads GG, Kagan A, Gordon T, Palesch Y. Alcohol and mortality: the Honolulu Heart Study. *Amer J Med.* 1980; 68(2):164-9.

15. Boaz NT. *Evolving Health: The Origins of Illness and How the Modern World is Making Us Sick.* New York, NY: John Wiley & Sons, 2002.

16. Boldsen JL. *Patterns of Advance Age Mortality in the Medieval Village Tirup.* Rostock, Germany: Max Planck Institute for Demographic Research, 1995.

17. Bortz W. *Dare to be 100: 99 Steps to a Long, Healthy Life.* New York, NY: Fireside, 1996.

18. Breslow L, Breslow N. Health practices and disability: Some evidence from Alameda County. *Prev Med.* 1993;22(1):86-95.

19. Buettner D. *The Blue Zones: Lessons for Living Longer from the People Who've Lived the Longest.* Washington, DC: National Geographic, 2009.

20. Butler RN, et al. Is there an antiaging medicine? *J Gerontol A Biol Sci Med Sci.* 2002:57(9):8333-8338.

21. Capurso A, et al. Epidemiological and socioeconomic aspects of Italian centenarians. *Arch Geron Geriat.* 1997;25(2):149-157.

22. Chan YC, Suzuki M, Yamamoto S. Nutritional status of centenarians assessed by activity and anthropometric, hematological, and biochemical characteristics. *J Nutr Sci Vitaminology.* 1997;43(1):73-81.

23. Church TS, et al. Cardiorespiratory fitness and body mass index as predictors of cardiovascular disease mortality among men with diabetes. *Arch Int Med.* 2005; 165:2114-2120.

24. Crose R. *Why Women Live Longer Than Men.* New York, NY: John Wiley & Sons, 1997.

25. Danaei G, et al. The preventable causes of death in the United States: Comparative risk assessment of dietary, lifestyle, and metabolic risk factors. *Pub Lib of Science Med.* 2009 Apr 28; 6(4): e1000058.

26. Danaei G, et al. The promise of prevention: The effects of four preventable risk factors on national life expectancy and life expectancy disparities by race and county in the United States. *Pub Lib of Science Med.* 2010 Mar 23; 7(3) e1000248.

27. Daviglus M, et al. Fish consumption and the 30-year risk of fatal myocardial infarction. *New Engl J Med.* 1997;336:1046-1053.

28. Denollet J, et al. Personality as independent predictor of long-term mortality in patients with coronary heart disease. *Lancet.* 1996;347:417-421.

29. Denollet J, et al. Type D Personality: A potential risk factor identified. *J Psychosom Res.* 2000;49:255-266.

30. Eskelinen MH, et al. Midlife coffee and tea drinking and the risk of late-life dementia: A population-based CAIDE study. *J Alzheimers Dis.* 2009;16(1):85-91.

31. Evert J, et al. Morbidity profiles of centenarians: survivors, delayers, and escapers. *J Gerontol A Biol Sci Med Sci.* 2003;58(3):232-237.

32. Fischer JG, et al. Dairy product intake of the oldest old. *J Amer Diet Ass.* 1995;95:918-921.

33. Flanigan RJ, Sawyer KF. *Longevity Made Simple: How to Add 20 Good Years to Your Life. Lessons from Decades of Research.* Denver, CO: Williams Clark Publishing, 2007.

34. Fraser GE. *Diet, Life Expectancy, and Chronic Disease: Studies of Seventh-day Adventists and Other Vegetarians.* New York, NY: Oxford University Press, 2003.

35. Galioto A, et al. Cardiovascular risk factors in centenarians. *Exp Gerontol.* 2008;43(2):106-113.

36. Gavrilov LA, Gavrilove NS. *The Biology of Life Span: A Quantitative Approach.* New York, NY: Harwood, 1991.

37. Goscienski PJ. *Health Secrets of the Stone Age: What We Can Learn from Deep in Prehistory to Become Leaner, Livelier, and Longer-Lived* (2nd Ed). Oceanside, CA: Better Life, 2005.

38. Grundy SM. Age as a risk factor: You are as old as your arteries. *Am J Cardiology.* 1999;83:1455-1457.

39. Hagberg B, et al. Cognitive functioning in centenarians: A coordinated analysis of results from three countries. *J Gerontol B. Psychol Sci Soc Sci.* 2001;56(3):P141-P151.

40. Harvard Medical School. *Living to 100: What's the secret?* Boston, MA: Harvard Health Publications, 2004.

41. Harvard Medical School. Putting the *joie de vivre* back into health: The eat-your-peas mode of staying healthy is changing to include chocolate, sleep, and a few other things most people enjoy. In: AL Komaroff (Ed.), *Harvard Health Letter.* 2009;34(6):1-3.

42. Harvard Medical School. The very old: How different from you and me? In AL Komaroff (Ed.). *Harvard Health Letter.* 2005;30(4):1-2.

43. Heilbronn LK, et al. Caloric restriction and aging: Review of the literature and implications for studies in humans. *Am J Clin Nutr.* 2003;78:361-369.

44. Hetzel L, Smith AD. *The 65 Years and Older Population: 2000.* Washington, DC: US Census Bureau, 2001. Publication C2KBR/01-10.

45. Hirose N, et al. Tokyo Centenarian Study. 4. Apolipoprotein E phenotype in Japanese centenarians living in the Tokyo Metropolitan Area. *Jap J Genetics.* 1997;34(4):267-70.

46. Howard M. *Achieving Generation C: 12 Steps to Make It to 100 Years Old.* Concord, CA: Biomed General, 2005.

47. Hu FB, et al. Fish and omega-3 fatty acid intake and risk of coronary heart disease in women. *JAMA.* 2002:287:1815-1821.

48. Jeune B. *Population Studies of Aging Number 15.* Odense, Denmark: Center for Health and Social Policy, Odense University, 1994.

49. Jeune B, Vaupel JW (Eds). *Exceptional Longevity: From Prehistory to the Present.* Vol 2. Odense, Denmark: Monographs on Population Aging 2, Odense University Press, 1995.

50. Kannisto V. *Development of oldest-old mortality, 1950-1990: Evidence from 28 developed countries.* Monographs on Population Aging, No. 1. Odense, Denmark: Odense University Press, 1994.

51. Kannisto V, et al. Reductions in mortality at advanced ages: Several decades of evidence from 27 countries. *Popul Devel Rev.* 1994;20(4):793-810.

52. Katan MB. Weight-loss diets for the prevention and treatment of obesity. *N Engl J Med.* 2009;360(9):923-925.

53. Klapcinska B, et al. Antioxidant defenses in centenarians (A preliminary study). *Acta Biochem Pol.* 2000;47(2):281-292.

54. Kotz D. *10 healthy habits that may help you live to 100.* U. S. News & World Report. *http://health.msn.com/print.aspx?cp-documentid=100233437&page=0.* Accessed January, 2010.

55. Kris-Etherton P, et al. Omega-3 fatty acids and cardiovascular disease: New recommendations from the American Heart Association. *Arterio Thromb Vasc Biol.* 2003;23:151-152.

56. LaLanne J. *Revitalize Your Life.* Fern Park, FL: Hastings House Publishers, 2003.

57. Lehr U. 100-years-old—A contribution on the research of longevity. *Zeitschrift Fur Gerontologie.* 1991;24(5):227-232.

58. Liebman B. You must remember this: How to keep your brain young. *Nutrition Action.* 2009;36(3):3-7.

59. Mahoney D, Restak R. *The Longevity Strategy: How to Live to 100 Using the Brain-Body Connection.* New York, NY: Wiley, 1999.

60. Manton KG, Vaupel, JW. Survival after the age of 80 in the United States, Sweden, France, England, and Japan. *N Engl J Med.* 1995;333:1232-1235.

61. Martin P, et al. Personality, life events and coping in the oldest old. *Int J Aging Hum Dev.* 1992;34(1):19-30.

62. Martin P, et al. Social and psychological resources of the oldest old. *Exp Aging Res.* 1996;22:121-139.

63. Masul, et al. Do personality characteristics predict longevity? Findings from the Tokyo Centenarian Study. *Age.* 2006;28(4):353-361.

64. Mecocci P, et al. Plasma antioxidants and longevity: A study on healthy centenarians. *Free Radical Biol Med.* 2000;28(8);1243-1248.

65. Messina M, Ho S, Alekel DL. Skeletal benefits of soy isoflavones: A review of the clinical trial and epidemiologic data. *Curr Opin Clin Nutr Metab Care.* 2004;7(6): 649-658.

66. Ming Wei, et al. Relationship between low cardiorespiratory fitness and mortality in normal-weight, overweight, and obese men. *JAMA.* 1999;282:1547-1553.

67. Morris M, et al. Consumption of fish and omega-3 fatty acids and risk of incident Alzheimer's disease. *Arch Neurol.* 2003;60:940-946.

68. Murphy R. *Baby boomers' guide to healthy aging.* Unpublished manuscript. 2003.

69. Murray CHL, et al. Eight Americas: Investigating mortality disparities across races, counties, and race-counties in the United States. *PLofS Med.* 2006;3(9):e260.

70. Murray CJ, Kulkami S, Ezzati M. Eight Americas: New perspectives on U. S. health disparities. *Am J Prev Med.* 2005 Dec 29 (5 Suppl): 4-10.

71. O'Brien M. *Successful Aging.* Concord, CA: Biomed General, 2005.

72. Olshansky SJ, Perls TT. New developments in the illegal provision of growth hormone for "anti-aging" and bodybuilding. *JAMA.* 2008;299(23):2792-2794.

73. Ozaki A, et al. The Japanese Centenarian Study: Autonomy was associated with health practices as well as physical status. *J Am Geriatr Soc.* 2006;55(1): 95-101.

74. Perls TT. Anti-aging quackery: Human growth hormone and tricks of the trade—more dangerous than ever. *J Gerontol A Biol Sci Med Sci.* 2004;59(7):682-691.

75. Perls TT. Centenarians prove the compression of morbidity hypothesis, but what about the rest of us who are genetically less fortunate? *Med Hypoth.* 1997;49:405-407.

76. Perls TT. Dementia-free centenarians. *Exper Gerontol.* 2004;39:1587-1593.

77. Perls TT. DHEA and testosterone in the elderly. *N Engl J Med.* 2007;356(6):636.

78. Perls TT. The different paths to 100. *Am J Clin Nutr.* 2006;83(2):484S-487S.

79. Perls TT. The oldest old. *Scientific American.* 1995;272(1):70-75.

80. Perls TT, et al. Life-long sustained mortality advantage of siblings of centenarians. *Proc Natl Acad Sci USA.* 2002;99(12):8442-8447.

81. Perls TT, Albert L, Fretts RC. Middle-aged mothers live longer. *Nature.* 1997;389:133.

82. Perls TT, Fretts RC. The evolution of menopause and human life span. *Ann Hum Biol.* 2001:28(3):237-245.

83. Perls TT, Morris JN, Ooi WL, Lipsitz LA. The relationship between age, gender and cognitive performance in the very old: The effect of selective survival. *J Am Geriatr Soc.* 1993;41(11):1193-1201.

84. Perls TT, Reisman NR, Olshansky SJ. Provision or distribution of growth hormone for "antiaging": Clinical and legal issues. *JAMA.* 2005;294(16):2086-2090.

85. Perls TT, Silver MH, Lauerman JF. *Living to 100: Lessons in Living to Your Maximum Potential at Any Age.* New York, NY: Basic Books, 1999.

86. Poon L, et al. The Georgia Centenarian Study. *Int J Aging Human Dev.* 1992;34(1):1-17.

87. Poon L, et al. *Who Will Survive to 105?* Chicago, IL: Encyclopedia Britannica, Inc., 1997.

88. Pratt S, Matthews K. *Superfoods Rx: Fourteen Foods That Will Change Your Life.* New York, NY: Harper, 2004.

89. Putnam RD. *Bowling Alone: The Collapse and Revival of American Community.* New York, NY: Simon and Schuster, 2001.

90. Regius O, Beregi E, Klinger A. Extended family, immediate family and caregiver contacts of 100-year-old patients in Hungary. *Zeitschrift Fur Gerontologie.* 1994;27(6): 456-458.

91. Robbins J. *Healthy at 100.* New York, NY: Random House, 2006.

92. Robine J-M, Allard M. *Jeanne Calment: Validation of the Duration of her Life.* Odense, Denmark: Validation of Exceptional Longevity, Odense University Press, 1999.

93. Robinson JG, Stone NJ. Antiatherosclerotic and antithrombotic effects of omega-3 fatty acids. *Am J Cardiol.* 2006;99:39i-49i.

94. Roizen MF, Oz MC. *You Staying Young: Owners Manual for Extending Your Warranty.* New York, NY: Free Press, 2007.

95. Ross PD, et al. A comparison of hip fractures among Native Japanese, Japanese Americans, and American Caucasians. *Am J Epidemiol.* 1991;133:801-809.

96. Rowe JW, Kahn RL. *Successful Aging.* New York, NY: Dell Publishing, 1999.

97. Sacks FM, et al. Comparison of weight-loss diets with different compositions of fat, protein, and carbohydrates. *N Engl J Med.* 2009;360(9):859-873.

98. Salim Y, et al. Effect of potentially modifiable risk factors associated with myocardial infarction in 52 countries (the INTERHEART Study): Case-Control Study. *Lancet.* 2004;364:937-952.

99. Sapolsky RM. *Why Zebras Don't Get Ulcers.* New York, NY: WH Freeman & Co, 1998.

100. Samuelsson SM, et al. The Swedish centenarian study: A multidisciplinary study of five consecutive cohorts at the age of 100. *Int J Aging Hum Dev.* 1997;45(3):223-253.

101. Schoenhofen EA, et al. Characteristics of 32 supercentenarians. *J Am Geriatr Soc.* 2006;54(8):1237-1240.

102. Sohal RS, et al. Oxidative stress, caloric restriction, and aging. *Science.* 1996;273:59-63.

103. Stern PC, Carstensen LL (Eds.). *The Aging Mind: Opportunities in Cognitive Research.* Washington, DC: National Academy Press, 2000.

104. Suzman RM, Willis DP, Manton KG. *The Oldest Old.* London, UK: Oxford University Press, 1992.

105. Terry DF, et al. Association of longer telomeres with better health in centenarians. *J Gerontol A Biol Sci Med Sci.* 2008;63(8):809-812.

106. Terry DF, et al. Cardiovascular delay in centenarian offspring. *J Gerontol A Biol Sci Med Sci.* 2004;59(4):385-389.

107. Terry DF, et al. Disentangling the roles of disability and morbidity in survival to exceptional old age. *Arch Int Med.* 2008;168(3):277-283.

108. Terry DF, et al. Lower all-cause, cardiovascular, and cancer mortality in centenarians' offspring. *J Am Geriatr Soc.* 2004;52(12):2074-2076.

109. Tourlouki E, et al. The 'secrets' of the long livers in Mediterranean islands: The MEDIS study. *Eur Jour Pub Health.* 2009; doi:10.1093/eurpub/ckp192.

110. Unger JB, et al. Variation in the impact of social network characteristics on physical functioning in elderly persons: MacArthur Studies of Successful Aging. *J Gerontol B Psychol Sci Soc Sci.* 1999;54(5):S245-S251.

111. Vaillant GE. *Aging Well: Surprising Guideposts to a Happier Life from the Landmark Harvard Study of Adult Development*. New York, NY: Little, Brown, 2003.

112. Vaupel JW, et al. Biodemographic trajectories of longevity. *Science*. 1998;280:855-859.

113. Vaupel JW, Jeune B. *The Emergence and Proliferation of Centenarians*. Rostock, Germany: Max Planck Institute for Demographic Research, 1995.

114. Walford R, Walford L. *The Anti-Aging Plan: The Nutrient-Rich, Low-Calorie Way of Eating for a Longer Life—The Only Diet Scientifically Proven to Extend Your Healthy Years*. New York, NY: Marlowe, 2005.

115. Weil A. *Healthy Aging: A Lifelong Guide to Your Physical and Spiritual Well-Being*. New York, NY: Alfred A. Knopf, 2005.

116. Whalley L. *The Aging Brain*. New York, NY: Columbia University Press, 2001.

117. Willcox BJ, Willcox DC, Suzuki M. *The Okinawa Program: How the World's Longest-Lived People Achieve Everlasting Health—and How You Can Too*. New York, NY: Clarkson Potter, Random House, 2001.

118. Willcox BJ, Willcox DC, Suzuki M. *The Okinawan Diet Plan: Get Leaner, Live Longer, and Never Feel Hungry*. New York, NY: Three Rivers Press, Random House, 2005.

119. Willcox BJ, et al. Siblings of Okinawan centenarians exhibit lifelong mortality advantages. *J Gerontol A Biol Sci Med Sci*. 2006;61:345-354.

120. Willcox BJ, et al. Substantial advantage for longevity in siblings of Okinawan centenarians. *Genetic Epidemiology*. 2005;29:286.

121. Willcox DC, et al. Caloric restriction and human longevity: What can we learn from the Okinawans? *Biogerontology*. 2006;7:173-177.

122. Willett WC. *Eat, Drink, and Be Healthy*. New York, NY: Free Press, 2001.

123. Wilmoth JR. *The Earliest Centenarians: A Statistical Analysis*. Rostock, Germany: Max Planck Institute for Demographic Research, 1995.

124. Zyczkowska J, et al. The prevalence of cardiovascular disease factors among centenarians is low: Risk factors in centenarians. *Eur J Cardiovasc Prev Rehabil*. 2006;13(6):993-995.

Internet References

1. AARP Andrus Foundation. *www.andrus.org*

2. Alliance for Aging Research. *www.agingresearch.com*

3. Alzheimer's Association. *www.alz.org*

4. American Association of Retired Persons (AARP). *www.aarp.org*

5. American Federation for Aging Research. *www.afar.org*

6. American Heart Association. *www.americanheart.org*

7. American Society on Aging. *www.asaging.org*

8. Georgia Centenarian Study.
   www.uga.edu/geron/research/centenarianstudy.php

9. Gerontology Research Group. *www.grg.org*

10. International Federation on Aging. *www.ifa-fiv.org*

11. National Center for Health Statistics (United States).
    www.cdc.gov/nchswww

12. National Institute on Aging. *www.nih.gov/nia*

13. National Weight Control Registry. *www.nwcr.ws*.

14. New England Centenarian Study. *www.bumc.bu.edu/centenarian*

15. Okinawan Centenarian Study. *www.okicent.org/study*

16. Supercentenarian Research Foundation. *www.grg.org*

17. The Living to 100 Life Expectancy Calculator. *www.livingto100.com*

NOTES:

May

NOTES: